# abortion

## A WORLDWIDE PERSPECTIVE

# abortion

## A WORLDWIDE PERSPECTIVE

Colin Francome
and
Marcel Vekemans

**Middlesex**
**University**
**PRESS**

First published in 2007 by Middlesex University Press

Copyright © Colin Francome

ISBN: 978 1 904750 23 9

A CIP catalogue record for this book is available from
The British Library

Design by Helen Taylor

Printed in the UK by Ashford Colour Press Ltd

Middlesex University Press
North London Business Park
Oakleigh Road South
London N11 1QS

Tel: +44 (0)20 8411 5734: +44 (0)20 8411 4162
Fax: +44 (0)20 8411 5736

www.mupress.co.uk

# ABORTION: A WORLDWIDE PERSPECTIVE

- According to the World Health Organization (WHO), the unsafe abortion rate per thousand women of fertile age is 16 in developing countries compared to two per thousand in the developed world.

- In this analysis we consider the evidence of 82 countries covering over 90 per cent of women and every country with more than 20 million people. What emerges is that unsafe abortion is largely a problem of poverty. Women in rich countries can have safe abortions locally and others can travel to countries where abortion is safe. In contrast, poor people have to face the hazards of abortion outside safe legal health services.

- Apart from the women who die there are numerous others who suffer morbidity. The World Health Organization estimates that around 20–30% of women having an unsafe abortion suffer reproductive tract infections and that around 2% become infertile.

- There are those following religious doctrine who believe abstinence is the answer to unwanted pregnancy. We have yet to find a society where this has proved successful. Consequently we propose good quality education, contraception and the right to choose a safe abortion service.

- The deaths of women occur disproportionately in poor countries. WHO estimated in 2000 that around 67,500 deaths occurred in developing countries while there were only around 300 in developed countries. Over 99% of abortion deaths were in developing countries.

- Official figures suggest four times as many die from unsafe abortion as are killed in terrorist attacks around the world. Yet while terrorism dominates the media, and billions are spent on prevention, unsafe abortion remains the silent killer.

# ACKNOWLEDGEMENTS

Special thanks to Stan Henshaw of the Guttmacher Institute who wrote most of the US chapter and commented on the other chapters.

Many others helped with this book. They included Margaret McGovern at the Family Planning Association; Evert Ketting; Wendy Savage of Doctors for a Woman's Choice on Abortion; Louise Bury, Tony Kerridge, Tim Black and Diana Thomas of Marie Stopes International; Elizabeth Rees for copy editing and general advice and Celia Cozens for continuous support from Middlesex University Press.

*Colin Francome*


IPPF's Regional Offices and Member Associations have over the years communicated to IPPF's Central Office many invaluable materials, data, statistics, and descriptions concerning the abortion issues in their region or country. Their inputs have been collected over time and have served now as important ground materials for this book.

*Marcel Vekemans*

# CONTENTS

# INTRODUCTION

*RESTRICTIVE LAWS DO NOT REDUCE*
*THE ABORTION RATE, THEY MERELY*
*RESULT IN WOMEN DYING.*

**Dr Dorothy Shaw 2006**

In the year 2000 there were an estimated 67,800 maternal deaths due to unsafe abortions. In 2005 there were a reported 14,602 deaths by terrorist attacks (WHO 2004: 13; Wright 2006: 509). Therefore over four times as many people died from unsafe abortion as were killed in all the terrorist attacks around the world. Yet while terrorism dominates the media and billions are spent on preventing terrorist attacks, unsafe abortion remains the silent killer. Furthermore, it is only part of the problem of unnecessary maternal deaths in childbirth. We write this book in the hope that governments can be encouraged to change their policies and provide all the women in the world with good quality care.

The deaths of women occur disproportionately in poor countries. Of the deaths an estimated 67,500 (99%) occurred in developing countries while there were only around 300 in developed countries. The unsafe abortion rate per thousand women of fertile age was 16 in developing countries and only two in developed ones. Therefore the rate was eight times higher in the poorer countries than the richer ones and unsafe abortion is largely a problem of poverty (WHO 2004: 13). Apart from the women who die there are numerous others who suffer morbidity. The WHO estimates that around 20–30% of women having an unsafe abortion suffer reproductive tract infections and that of these infections 20–40% lead to upper genital tract infections. The result is that around 2% of women become infertile because of unsafe abortion and 5% suffer chronic infection (Grimes et al. 2006). Each year around 510,000 women around the world die from pregnancy-related causes: the level of unnecessary deaths is clearly an important issue.

Legal abortion is now available in all industrialised countries except Ireland, Malta and Poland, and in many developing countries including the most populous – China and India. National health insurance also covers the procedure in most industrialised countries. Abortion is still highly restricted in most countries of Latin America and Africa and in parts of Asia. Worldwide, the trend toward relaxing restrictions has continued. In the past few years, restrictions have been reduced in Colombia, Ethiopia, Nepal, Switzerland, Portugal and Mexico City.

## Abortion is a reality

The evidence presented in this book will show that abortion cannot be eliminated by authorities prohibiting it. Governments can only determine whether abortions are safe and legal or unsafe and illegal. We will see that in countries like the United States and Britain a great number of abortions occurred even when abortion was illegal. Dorothy Shaw, president of the International Federation of Gynecology and Obstetrics (FIGO), speaking at a WHO forum in December 2006 stated that evidence on sexual and reproductive health 'clearly shows the continuing track record of preventable deaths and illness in catastrophic numbers that would not be tolerated in most other imaginable situations'. She continued to say those sexual and reproductive rights are integral parts of basic human rights and that 'restrictive laws do not reduce the abortion rate they merely result in women dying' (WHO Forum 2006).

It is relatively rare for countries to legalise abortion and subsequently make it illegal. Romania, however, provides an example of the problems that can follow this. In 1965 it had a birth rate of 14.6 per thousand population and 64 abortion deaths. In 1966 it restricted abortion rights and access to contraception. The birth rate almost doubled to 27.4 in 1967 and the number of abortion deaths rose to 170, almost three times the 1965 level. In subsequent years the number of abortion deaths rose to 364 in 1971, over five times the earlier level, and the birth rate in that year was down to 19.1 and approaching its earlier level (Francome 1976).

If abortion is not readily and legally accessible, poorer women will be forced to seek treatment from local operators with potentially disastrous results. Richer women, however, will become abortion tourists. In the early part of the twentieth century British women went to France for abortions. When the British law was changed French women began travelling to Britain in great numbers. In the early 1960s Swedish women went to Poland and women from the USA went to Britain. After legalisation in New York in 1970, Canadian women went to the USA. When financial restrictions were placed on poorer women in the USA they began going to Mexico. German and Belgian women went to Holland until their laws changed. In Britain in 1972 over 50,000 women from overseas had abortions in the country and there was a spectacular growth in the number of Spanish women until Spain's law changed. In 2006 Swedish operators expressed a willingness to help their Polish neighbours who had earlier helped their own women obtain treatment. Irish women still travel to Britain even from the North where the 1967 Abortion Act does not apply. Over the years there have been distinct patterns where women travel abroad for abortions but simultaneously activists are working to change the law in their home country.

The International Conference on Population and Development (ICPD) of 1994 drew attention to the high levels of maternal mortality and a target was set to halve the 1990 rates by the year 2000 and halve it again by the year 2015. Far more resources will be needed as well as legalisation of abortion if the maternal mortality rates are to achieve these substantial reductions (UN 2004).

## Need for worldwide change

As recently as the 1960s there were only a few places in the world, such as the Soviet Union, which had liberal abortion laws. When the British Abortion Act 1967 took effect on 27 April 1968, with no residential requirement, it allowed rich women from all over the world to have access to safe legal abortions. This was followed by great change in laws in other countries. In the period up to 1982, 12 countries passed laws to allow abortion on request. These were Austria, Denmark, France, German Democratic Republic, Italy, the Netherlands, Norway, Singapore, Slovenia, Sweden, Tunisia, the USA and Yugoslavia.

In addition, 26 countries extended grounds for abortion but did not officially give the right to choose. These were Australia, Belize, Canada, Chile, Cyprus, El Salvador, Fiji, Finland, German Federal Republic, Greece, Guatemala, Hong Kong, Iceland, India, Israel, Korea (Republic of), Kuwait, Luxembourg, Morocco, New Zealand, Peru, Seychelles, South Africa, United Arab Emirates and Zimbabwe. Chile and El Salvador have since eliminated all grounds for abortion and so move in the opposite direction.

Those countries providing women with the right to choose, or at least abortion on a wide variety of grounds, were predominantly the richer countries. In recent years there have been further changes. In 1995 the Beijing Platform for Action called on governments to rescind restrictive abortion laws that punish women, and from then until June 2007 the following countries liberalised their laws: Albania (1996), Benin (2003), Bhutan (2004) Burkina Faso (1996), Cambodia (1997), Chad (2002), Columbia (2006), Ethiopia (2004), Guinea (2000), Guyana (1995), Mali (2002), Nepal (2002), Portugal

(2007), St Lucia (2004), South Africa (1996), Swaziland (2005), Switzerland (2002) and Togo (2007) (Katzive 2007). In April 2007 Mexico City passed a law allowing abortion on request in the early part of pregnancy.

## Children born into poverty

There is a very high correlation with large family size and child poverty. Niger is a good example. The United Nations (UN) reports that the country had the highest fertility rate in the world at 7.9 children per woman (2005). It also has high infant mortality at 153 per thousand in 2005. This means that for every 100 fertile women in the country an average of 110 infants die before the age of 1. Others will die later in childhood. The suffering this waste of life causes can only be imagined, as women and their partners are clearly not able to care for their children adequately. Furthermore, there will be many other children who survive but do so without proper nutrition or health and social care. The introduction of facilities for contraception and abortion, especially as part of a wider programme to improve medical and social support, could prevent much misery amongst these women who have to give birth to children for whom they cannot adequately care.

Other countries are in a similar position. Women in Timor-Leste, Afghanistan, Guinea-Bissau and Uganda all had an average family size of over seven children per woman during the period 2000–2005. Other countries such as Mali, Burundi, Liberia, Angola and the Democratic Republic of Congo had a fertility rate of over six children per woman. All these also have high rates of ill health amongst both women and children. Overall in the poor countries 170 million children are underweight and over 3 million of these children die each year as a result (Wright 2006: 485). Access to modern contraceptives and abortion facilities are part of a wider need to improve maternal and child health.

## International developments in aid for family planning

Official Norwegian development assistance started in 1952 and emphasis on family planning assistance began in 1966. Experts pointed out that population growth was hampering economic growth. In 1968 the Norwegian parliament decided that family planning should be a priority for development assistance. Norad, the government development agency, allocated 10% of bilateral development assistance to family planning in 1970. In the following year parliament supported Norad's policy proposal of placing family planning within primary care with the aim of helping to improve the health of women and their children (Austveg and Sundby 2005). The importance of contraception and reproductive health to development was also recognised in 1989 at a conference in Amsterdam, which placed as a target developed countries providing 4% of their overseas development aid to population activities (de Bruijn and Horstman 2005).

At the International Conference on Population and Development (ICPD) in 1994, Norway produced a report emphasising 'the seriousness of present population growth and the need to counteract the negative effects on the environment'. According to Population Action International, Norway was the only country before 1994 to allocate at least 4% of overseas development assistance to population. Norway has been one of the largest donors to the United Nations Population Fund (UNPFA) since its inception in 1969 and also a large donor to the International Planned Parenthood Federation (IPPF). Overall the proportion of family planning aid in 2004 from all donors was 5.5% and therefore the 1994 target has been achieved. However, in that year in several countries the percentage was below 2%: these were Austria (0.5%), Italy (1.0%), Greece (1.4%), Spain (1.5%) and Germany (1.9%). Improved contributions from these countries would be useful in an area where funds are short. Countries above the 5% level included the Netherlands (10.2%), the USA (9.2%), the UK (8.4%) and Sweden (7.2%) (Secretary General 2005).

The 1994 ICPD in Cairo led to the first major international agreement on unsafe abortion with 180 countries agreeing a programme of action. Its proposals fell short of making the decision that a woman should have the right to decide whether to terminate a pregnancy in the early months, but it called attention to the public impact of unsafe abortion and the need to expand family planning services to reduce recourse to abortion. In paragraph 7.2 it stated:

> Reproductive rights ... rest on the recognition of the basic right of all couples and individuals to decide freely and responsibly the number, spacing and timing of their children and to have the information and means to do so, and the right to attain the highest standard of sexual and reproductive health. It also includes their right to make decisions concerning reproduction free of discrimination, coercion and violence, as expressed in human rights documents (Hessini 2005).

Hessini assessed how the principles and recommendations of the conference have been applied to increasing women's access to 'affordable, safe and legal abortion services' in the decade up to 2004. The article suggested that studies have increased the knowledge of the magnitude of unsafe abortion, have raised the awareness of women's experience of illegal abortion, and linked it to other public health and women's rights issues. It drew attention to the fact that that there have been several studies of abortion complications. For example, one study estimated that over 20,000 women are being treated for abortion-related illness in Kenyan public hospitals. We will be providing similar evidence from a variety of countries.

It also stated that women still face numerous barriers in countries where abortion is legal. For example, in India where abortion has been legal for over 30 years, 76% of facilities were not licensed and 68% of providers were not registered. The quality of services can vary: a study in Tamil Nadu found that close to 30% of women seeking legal abortions experienced moderate to serious post-abortion complications. There is evidence of improvement since that time and the quality of care in India seems to be improving as we will discuss.

The overall response to the Cairo conference has been inadequate.    Observers comment: 'If spending on population and AIDS activities is completely in line with health in general, then it is safe to assume that consumers in developed countries pay more than half the burden of population and AIDS expenditures. Out of pocket spending by consumers especially the poor has important implications for policy initiatives aimed at reducing poverty' (RF News 2004). In 2005 an estimated 2.8 million people were estimated to have died from AIDS and 4.1 million to have been newly infected (Wright 2006: 490). While it is clearly right that resources should be provided in this area, this should not be at the expense of reproductive health.

The Millennium Development Goals grew out of the United Nations Millennium Declaration adopted by 189 member states in 2000. There were eight goals. Three of them were directly related to reproductive health. As mentioned earlier, it aimed to reduce the maternal mortality ratio by three-quarters and the under-5 mortality rate of children by two-thirds between 1990 and 2015. A third goal was to have halted the spread of AIDS and begun to reverse it by the year 2015. Other goals were to eradicate extreme poverty and hunger, promote gender equality and empower women, and ensure environment sustainability.

At the 2005 World Summit, leaders committed themselves to 'achieving universal access to reproductive health by 2015' as set out by ICPD. This aim was to be integrated into strategies to attain the internationally agreed development goals including those contained in the millennial declaration aimed at reducing maternal mortality, improving maternal health, reducing child mortality, improving gender equality, combating HIV/AIDS and eradicating poverty (RF News 2007). If this occurs we would expect the number of unsafe abortions to be reduced.

## The USA gag rule

A barrier to effective family planning assistance is a US policy that critics call the 'global gag rule' (the Mexico City policy). Under this rule, foreign non-governmental organisations which receive US family planning assistance are denied the right to use their own non-US funds to engage in abortion-related public policy debates, or perform legal abortions in cases other than a threat to the life of the woman, rape or incest. They are also not allowed to provide counselling or referral for abortion or to lobby to make abortion legal or more available. US funds can however be used for post-abortion care and for participating in scientific conferences about abortion. The global gag rule was reinstated by President George W Bush on his first day in office in January 2001 (Fisher 2005).

## World fertility rates

The world fertility rate has been declining. In 1970–1975 it was 4.5 children per woman. This had declined to 3.0 in 1990–1995 and then to 2.8 from 1995–2000. In the more developed regions fertility has been much lower than average. In the years 1970–1975 it was 2.1 children per woman but had declined to 1.6 in the period 1995–2000. In the less developed regions fertility was 5.4 children per woman in 1970–1975 and had declined by over two children a woman by 1995–2000 when the average had reduced to 3.1 children per woman. However, it is the poorest women who have the highest birth rate. In the countries designated by the UN as the least developed regions the birth rate has not fallen so fast. In 1970–1975 it was 6.6 children per woman and had declined by one child per woman to 5.5 in 1995–2000. More children are therefore born to those women in poverty where there are higher rates of infant deaths (UN 2004: 29).

Within these overall figures there are some countries which have greatly decreased their birth rate. In Iran there were an average of 6.4 children per woman in 1964 but by 1996 it had reduced by nearly four children to 2.5 per woman. Similarly, in Brazil the average woman had 5.7 children in 1965 and the number fell to 2.3 in 1996 (UN 2004). Therefore rapid changes can occur and it is feasible that poor countries could make immense strides in a short time.

## Contraception

Worldwide contraceptive use by married or cohabiting women was reported by the UN to be 62% in 1997. The most common method was sterilisation which was used by one in five (20%); a further one in 25 (4%) used vasectomy. Around one in seven (15%)

used the intra-uterine device and one in 12 (8%) used oral contraception. Condom usage was only one in 20 (5%) (these figures were based on the responses of women and it could be that single men made greater use of the condom). Fewer than 3% were using injection methods and 1% vaginal foam. These methods are known as modern methods. In addition 3% used withdrawal and just under 3% the rhythm method (UN 2004).

Worldwide, fewer than a quarter of couples were using male methods of contraception. Researchers may subdivide the male contribution as participatory (condom, vasectomy) and co-operative (withdrawal, rhythm) (UN 2004: 59).

Around one in five women have an unmet need for contraception where they have problems of access. At the 21st special session of the General Assembly of the UN, targets were set to reduce this unmet need by 75% in 2010 and 100% by 2050.

## Costs of restrictive laws

Hessini drew attention to the fact that restrictive laws, unsafe abortions and poor standards of care lead to higher costs in some respects. Using data from Africa, a model showed that treating incomplete abortions in hospitals costs around ten times the cost of providing safe legal abortions in a primary health centre. Costs are also reduced where manual vacuum aspiration (MVA) is used instead of dilation and curettage (D&C). In 1995 the Fourth World Conference on Women called for governments to 'review laws containing punitive measures against women who have undergone illegal abortions'.

There have been a number of other important events including a 2003 conference in Ethiopia discussing unsafe abortion in Africa and in 2004 a South African conference on the role of medical abortion in expanding women's access to safe treatment (Hessini 2005: 91).

International organisations have also taken an increased role. One such is the Committee on the Elimination of Discrimination against Women (CEDAW). This group points out that neglecting health care that only women need is a form of sex discrimination which governments are obliged to remedy.

## Abortion as a controversial issue

Passions often run high when debating the issue. Those of us who support the woman's right to choose point to the dangers of illegal abortion. We also draw attention to the fact that if women are forced to bear children they cannot look after properly, it can lead to social problems. Opponents of choice may point to the rights of the fetus to be born and argue that life begins at the moment of conception. They may also argue that legalising abortion may lead to a decline in morals. This book will agree strongly with the view put forward in Boston, USA, by the Roman Catholic priest Robert Drinan. This is that the fact that some people believe abortion to be wrong should not impinge on the quality of care for those who do not share that view (Francome 1984a: 112–13).

## Major religions and abortion

In the year 2000 Christians made up just under a third (32.8%) of the world's population with just over one in six (17.3%) people worldwide being Roman Catholic and 3.4% being Orthodox. Muslims made up just under one in five (19.9%) and they were divided between Shiite and Sunni Muslims. The third biggest grouping was the Hindus which consisted of around one in seven (13.3%) of the world's population. Other major religions were Buddhism (5.9%), Sikhism (0.4%) and Judaism (0.2%). Around one in eight people (12.6%) belonged to other religions or were non-religious (12.4%). In addition there were 2.4% avowed atheists (Smith 2003). Within each religious group there are likely to be those who are simply nominal members and also a variety of subgroups. Below we make observations on the attitudes to contraception and abortion of some major religious groups. However, few members of each group may follow the official teachings. This is particularly true of Roman Catholicism where few adherents follow the Pope in opposing artificial birth control or the Church's rigid attitudes to abortion.

## Jewish law

Although Jews make up a small proportion of the world's population, their religion greatly influenced the development of Christianity and Islam. The religion is subdivided into three main groupings – orthodox, conservative and reform – and within these there are myriad subdivisions. In some ways the orthodox are the most prescriptive in that they have a coherent long-standing belief system. Adherents should not have sexual intercourse until 12 days after the start of their menstrual period. Those with knowledge of the safe period will see this as a recipe for fertility. Furthermore, when the time in the month is right the man is obliged to copulate with his wife, and sex is regarded as a mikvah – a blessing. After women have a menstrual period they are regarded as unclean until they have had a ritual bath. Adherents are not allowed to work on the Sabbath, but if they put tall masts around the area it is designated an *eruv* and this allows them to carry out a wider range of activities.

The orthodox are not permitted to use contraception. Judaism does not recognise the fetus as being of equal status to the woman until its head is born. Once this has occurred 'the baby's life is considered equal to the mother's, and we may not choose one life over another' (Eisenberg 2007). However, in the womb the life of the fetus is subordinate to that of the mother and may be sacrificed 'if there is a direct threat to the life of the mother by carrying the fetus to term or through the act of childbirth, in such circumstance, the baby is considered tantamount to *rodef*, a pursuer after the mother with the intent to kill her' (Eisenberg 2007).

According to Eisenberg, Judaism recognises psychiatric as well as physical factors as potentially posing a threat to the life of the woman. Rabbi Waldenberg would allow an abortion of a fetus with deformity that would cause it to suffer in the first trimester and the termination of a fetus with a lethal defect such as Tay-Sachs disease up to the seventh month of gestation. The only reference to abortion in the Bible is in Exodus (21:22) where it says that if a man 'hurt a woman with child so that her fruit depart from her, and yet no mischief follow: he shall be surely punished according as the woman's husband will lay upon him'. Thus if the woman recovers it is seen as a minor event but if the woman dies then it would be a case of 'life for life'.

We shall see that in the Roman Catholic and Muslim religions there has been a debate as to when life begins. The Bible says: 'God formed man of the dust of the ground and breathed into his nostrils the breath of life and man became a living soul' (Genesis 2:7). From this it seems that life begins at birth and this ties in with the forgoing; but it seems sometimes the Bible implies that life begins later than birth. In Numbers (3:15) it is said that a census should number a male child only from the age of 1 month. Similarly in Leviticus (27:6) it seems that only children who have reached the age of 1 month should have a monetary value (Halperin 2007).

# Christianity

The largest world religion is Christianity. It began as a religion that was opposed to rules. Although Jesus was Jewish he often broke the rules that the religion imposed such as that he should not have healed on the Sabbath which would be regarded as work: the Bible tells he healed a man with a withered hand. Over the years the various churches and sects imposed various rules especially in the area of fertility, as we shall see. Christianity divided at an early stage into many different groups. The main division was between the Orthodox (Greek and Russian) and the Roman Catholic versions of Christianity. Both groups enjoined restrictions on the sexuality of the clergy. The Roman Catholic Church taught that all priests should be celibate but the Greek Orthodox Church only asked this of its higher clergy such as bishops.

## *The Roman Catholic Church and abortion*

Until 1869, apart from the three-year period 1588–1591, the Church held to a theory derived from Aristotle that a soul did not enter the male until 40 days after conception nor the female until 80 days after conception. Abortion could be carried out up to this time. As sex could not be determined it would not be difficult to argue for abortion up to 80 days or nearly three months' gestation. The *Catholic Encyclopaedia* published in 1913 explained that Aristotle's proposal had allowed abortion at the beginning of pregnancy and commented: 'The authority of his great name and the want of definite knowledge to the contrary caused this theory to be generally accepted up to recent times.' There is also evidence of an indulgent attitude towards birth control. A French bishop wrote to the Pope about a problem he was having with young married men using withdrawal as a method of contraception. He also found it difficult to convince a husband 'that he is to be considered in a condition of mortal sin unless he either lives chaste in marriage, or runs the risk of having an unlimited family' (Francome 1984a). In its reply (8 June 1842) the Holy See took a very gentle approach to the problem. It said that priests should not interrogate the men and if the wife should confess the fact they should 'deal with it in the most tender manner' (Francome 1984a: 24).

Things changed in the Church and one of the problems was a belief stated clearly in the British Catholic newspaper *The Universe* (22 May 1936) that 'it is now, and always has been, the mind of the Church that unbaptised infants go to Hell'. Owing to this belief during the period from 1869 until around the 1950s the Catholic Church took the view that abortion should not even be allowed to save the life of the woman. In the book *Moral Problems for Catholic Nurses* which was published with papal approval and in its fifth edition in 1935, it was stated that men often had to die in wars and similarly:

> A parallel case is the situation of a woman in a difficult labour, when her life and that of her unborn child are in extreme danger. In this situation it is the mother's duty to die rather than to consent to the killing of her child … better that ten thousand mothers should die than one fetus is unjustly killed (Finney 1935: 46).

One of the causes of the death of the woman was the attitude to pregnancies which occurred in the fallopian tubes (ectopic pregnancy). There is no possibility the pregnancy can go to term and so it would seem logical that the tube should be removed. However, as the *Catholic Encyclopaedia* explains, the Church decided on 20 March 1902 that an abortion in this case was not lawful. Similarly in 1935 Finney asked: 'If a surgeon, operating … discovers an ectopic fetus not yet viable, is it lawful for him to remove it?'

He continued: 'No it is not' (Finney 1935: 14).

In the years after the Second World War the Church changed its attitude and its leaders seemed to forget its earlier stance. In 1963 Britain's leading Catholic layman, Norman St John Stevas, said that the Catholic Church had never objected to an abortion for ectopic pregnancy (1963: 40). We have seen that the evidence does not support that statement. We shall see that in Chile, even in recent years, women have been forced to continue an ectopic pregnancy until it becomes life-threatening. At one stage women were obliged to die. Now some places merely insist treatment is delayed.

Some people style themselves 'pro life'. However, sometimes when restrictive Catholic doctrine is written into law it prevents women becoming mothers. Strict Church teaching opposes artificial insemination by donor and in 2007 a Church-inspired restrictive law caused the closure of the Novum clinic in Warsaw. This had been providing in vitro fertilisation, where Beata Skolimoska, who was 14 weeks pregnant and waiting for a check-up, commented that she was a 'believer in the Catholic Church' but that she was 'very frustrated by the religious policy adopted by the Government. I wanted to try the clinic again for a second child.' Reporters stated that at the clinic it was a man who was the most anguished; he could not believe that people should deny him and his wife the chance of having a baby (Perlez 2007).

Prenatal screening, with the option of abortion if the pregnancy becomes problematic, has allowed couples to try for a baby. For example, each child of couples who are carriers of Tay-Sachs disease has a 25% chance of having a genetic abnormality that causes death by the age of 5. With prenatal testing and abortion, these couples can have a full and healthy family and avoid having a child who would inevitably die at an early age. Without the availability of prenatal testing and termination many such couples would choose not to have children.

## Other Christian groups

The Methodists were among the first religious groups to support contraception in Britain and then to support the liberalisation of abortion. Lord Soper, the Methodist life peer, was a vocal supporter and the Methodist Conference called for liberalisation in 1966. The Church of England was more ambivalent. However, the Church Assembly Board of Social Responsibility passed a resolution to liberalise the law in 1965. Other groups to pass a resolution in favour of the Abortion Bill were the Congregationalist Church, the Church of Scotland, the Free Church Federal Council and the British Council of Churches (Francome 1984a: 87).

In the USA, the conservative Baptist communities tend to oppose abortion and there was at one time a so-called 'moral majority'. This was formed by Jerry Falwell in 1979. Richard Viquerie wrote in *The New Right* (1981): 'There are an estimated 85 million Americans, 50 million born again Protestants, 30 million morally Conservative Catholics, 3 million Mormons and 2 million Orthodox and Conservative Jews with whom to build a pro family, Bible believing coalition.' One of the weaknesses of this assessment is that it is not a majority but rather a third of the US population. Also, not all the morally conservative groups oppose abortion. The Seventh Day Adventists, for example, take issue with the anti-abortionists. KD Paulson, writing on the group's position, commented that the Adventists refused to criticise abortion in the same way as other Christian conservatives and opposed Christians who try to persuade governments to make it illegal. He commented that the ancient Egyptians condoned abortion and that one papyrus lists information as to how to induce one. He also argued that abortion did not arrive with legalisation but that in the 1920s one-quarter of pregnancies ended in a termination. He commented that making abortion illegal was ineffective, and as an example drew attention to the fact that from 1948 to 1958, 32 people were accused of abortion in Massachusetts and not one was convicted. He was vitriolic about the violence against abortion clinics in the USA and said it revealed 'the satanic spirit behind much of the so called "Pro Life" movement' (Paulson 2007).

## Islam

There is scope for wide variation in beliefs as the Koran does not mention abortion. The majority of orthodox Muslims in recent centuries permitted abortion up to the end of four months' gestation owing to a belief that the soul enters the fetus at this time. The Republic of Egypt produced a pamphlet entitled *Islam's Attitude toward Family Planning* in which it says: 'Jurists of the Shiite Zaidiva believe in the total permissibility of abortion before life is breathed into the fetus, no matter whether there is a justifiable excuse or not.' The Iranian Grand Ayatollah Y Saanei commented: 'If there are serious problems God sometimes does not require his creatures to practice his law. So under some conditions – such as parents' poverty or over-population – then abortion is allowed.' (*LA Times* 29 Dec 2000).

Other Muslims take the view that 'abortion does not abruptly become prohibited at a certain stage, but becomes increasingly disfavoured as the fetus develops' (personal communication). This belief has allowed the development of manual vacuum aspiration in Muslim countries. It is this procedure which we shall see has reduced the number of unsafe operations in Bangladesh.

## Other religions

The other large religions are Hinduism, Buddhism and Sikhism. Hinduism is the oldest of the world's major religions. It originated in India and spread to Nepal and Southeast Asia. It is a tolerant religion and accepts that other belief systems such as Christianity or Islam have value. It has the belief that individuals should connect themselves to the *Brahman* or Godhead. This is the spiritual source of the tangible universe (Wright 2006: 494). They also believe in reincarnation with one's subsequent status being dependent on one's actions. The cycle of reincarnation is ended when one obtains liberation from the finite world through self-discovery.

Buddhism was established by S Gautama (c.563–483 BC) who was born into Hinduism. At the age of 29 he left his wife and young son to seek enlightenment. The Buddha means 'the enlightened one' and the belief is that those who become enlightened pass into nirvana in which 'ideas and consciousness cease to be'. There are about 350 million Buddhists in 92 countries (Wright 2006: 496). On abortion they believe the woman must make the decision herself (Childbirth by Choice Trust 2007).

The Sikh religion was founded by Guru Nanak in the sixteenth century and advocates a search for eternal truth. It has around 19 million adherents worldwide, nearly all of whom live in or originate from the Punjab region of India. Sikhs believe that the woman's right far outweighs the right of the embryo or fetus, which is not given the status of a human person (Childbirth by Choice Trust 2007).

## Medical developments

One important development is that of manual vacuum aspiration. This makes use of a simple syringe with a plunger to generate the necessary pressure for uterine evacuation and plastic canulas of varying sizes. The amount of negative pressure obtained with manual vacuum aspiration is similar to that generated with a large, expensive electrical pump. Thus it can be used in low cost settings and after use can be sterilised or disinfected to be used again (Grimes et al. 2006).

An important innovation is that of medical abortion. Marge Berer writes:

> Medical abortion is the use of pills to cause a miscarriage. It represents a particularly important advance in abortion technology because it brings women's access to safe abortion closer to home … Medical abortion has been shown to be safe for over 15 years now, and as the word of its existence has spread, women all over the world have been using it, including in remote parts of developing countries (2005).

The British Medical Association explained that the woman usually takes mifepristone (RU 486); this blocks hormones which allow a pregnancy to continue. Two days later the woman takes a prostaglandin (misoprostol), which makes the uterus expel the fetus. The WHO recommends the combined use of mifepristone and misoprostol as being better than either one alone. Misoprostol was first used as a drug to prevent and cure ulcers and it is relatively cheap and available (Grimes et al. 2006). Women take the mifepristone tablet by mouth, and the misoprostol tablets are inserted vaginally or taken by mouth. This vaginal insertion can be effected by the woman, her partner or the provider. Women having such an abortion 'do not need a hospital bed in fact they don't need a bed at all' (Berer 2005a: 8).

By 2005 more than 22 million women in China, 1 million in France and around 3 million in the rest of the world had had a medical abortions and found it safe. In some areas of Norway it is now offered as the main abortion method and women have to request a different method if that is their choice. In Scotland in 2005 three in five (59%) abortions were medical. In England and Wales it was below half this figure (24%) (BMA 2007). Medical abortion has also grown in popularity in India. It is also suggested by observers that in areas of the world where there are restrictions on legal abortion, such as Africa, Latin America and some parts of Asia, misoprostol has been increasingly self-administered by women as an alternative to much less safe methods. Observers in Latin America in 2005 commented: 'Interest in the use of medical abortion has been growing during the past decade throughout Latin America using mainly misoprostol' (Lafaurie et al. 2005). Such self-administration led to the drug being banned in Brazil, which we shall see served only to create a black market and drive up the price. Indeed, observers suggest that the self-administration of misoprostol during the period 2000 to 2005 led to a reduction in maternal deaths due to abortion in both Brazil and Peru, and a review of death certificates in an urban area of Mexico found no deaths due to first trimester abortion 'perhaps in part because of the increasing use of medical methods (Lafaurie et al. 2005: 76). An in-depth study of 49 women who had medical abortions found that many women were happy with the lack of disruption to their lives. A 27-year-old government office administrator in Colombia said:

> The advantage is that you can go on normally with your life … While I was going through this I went to work like always. I just had to be careful about the bleeding, just like when you have a heavy period … Normal, it's totally normal, you just go on with your life as you normally would.

In this study cramps were the most common side-effect, reported by 46 of the 49 women. These were described as very strong by 17 women. Respondents pointed out that the most intense pain lasted two or three hours. However, in this study they were not following the World Health Organization guidelines (Lafaurie et al. 2005: 79).

Another development that has had some impact on safe abortion is the provision of contraceptive information to those who are in contact with the health services either to gain an abortion or to be treated for the after-effects of an unsafe operation. Research in Zimbabwe found that when contraceptive services were provided it reduced the number of future unwanted pregnancies by 50% (Grimes et al. 2006).

## Structure of the book

In this book we analyse the situation in all countries for which information is available and which have populations of over 20 million; this will cover over 90% of the world's population. We have also included a number of smaller countries where there is special interest, for example Israel as the only country with a majority of people of the Jewish religion and Ireland as a country with strong Roman Catholic links and an anti-abortion statement in its constitution. We use the United Nations classification of continents and consider them in alphabetical order. In considering each country we aim to provide some basic facts about the country, followed by a discussion of contraception and abortion. One of the questions we have considered is whether there is any society in the world which has been able to successfully convince its population to abstain from premarital sexuality, or alternatively, in countries where such attempts are made and contraception is not encouraged and abortion largely illegal, whether it leads rather to unsafe operations or women becoming sexual tourists. We draw conclusions from our findings in the final chapter.

# EUROPE

*THE RHYTHM METHOD WAS NO GOOD FOR YOUNG CZECHS. THEY DIDN'T WANT TO HAVE SEX ACCORDING TO A CALENDAR. THEY WANTED TO HAVE SEX WHEN THEIR PARENTS WEREN'T HOME.*

**Radim Uzel personal communication 2005**

The population of Europe was estimated at 140 million in 1750. It grew to 401 million by 1900, almost a tripling in size. During the nineteenth century, population grew rapidly in all European countries except France, Spain and Ireland. In Britain the population multiplied three and a half times between 1801, when the first census was taken, and 1900. In the period 1970 to 1975 the average woman had 2.2 children. This figure fell to 1.6 children per woman in the period 1990 to 1995 and to 1.4 from 1995–2000 (UN 2004: 29). Europe's population growth has reduced to well below replacement level in recent years.

The UN (2004) set out the abortion rate per thousand women aged 15–44 for the year 1999 (unless otherwise stated) in European countries as follows:

- **Eastern Europe**   Belarus (58), Bulgaria (43), Czech Republic (17), Hungary (31), Republic of Moldova (27), Poland, Romania (52), Russian Federation (62), Slovakia (1998:21), Ukraine (45)
- **Northern Europe**   Denmark (15), Estonia (48), Finland (11), Iceland (15), Ireland, Latvia (34), Lithuania (23), Norway (15), Sweden (18), United Kingdom (15)
- **Southern Europe**   Albania (22), Bosnia and Herzegovina, Croatia (15), Greece, Italy (11), Portugal, Slovenia (20), Spain (n/a)
- **Western Europe**   Austria, Belgium (6), France (13), Germany (8), Netherlands (1998:7) Switzerland (n/a)

There are still marked differences in social patterns between Eastern and Western Europe with Eastern European societies using less contraception and having much higher abortion rates: Russian women had ten times the rate of abortion as those in Belgium. Sociologists have noted that in the past Western European marriage differed from that in Eastern Europe in at least two main ways: first, Western Europe had a high average age of marriage and second, it had a high proportion who never married. Stone states that this is a unique feature of North-west European civilisation and lacks a satisfactory explanation (1977). In 1900 the Western European pattern of marriage extended broadly to the west of a line running from St Petersburg to Trieste. If we consider a selection of countries from the West of Europe there is a pattern: Austria, Germany, Great Britain, Holland, Italy and Sweden each had at least 60% of its women single in the age group 20–24 years and at least one in ten of its women were single in the age group 45–49 years; in contrast, in Hungary, Romania, Bulgaria, Serbia and Greece women married earlier and in each case the majority of the 20–24 age group were married. In Serbia, for example, 84% of women aged 20–24 were married. Furthermore, in Serbia only 1% of women were single in the age group 45–49 years, in Bulgaria 2%, in Romania 3% and in Hungary and Greece 4%. With young marriages there were other differences such as their often having being arranged by the parents (Hajnal 1965).

In Eastern Europe younger women aged 15–29 provide 83% of the births while in Western Europe only 63% (UN 2004: 34). The UN reported in 2004 that there were several European countries where the average age of marriage for women was above 30: Finland, France, Iceland, Ireland, Norway and Sweden.

The World Health Organization (WHO) reports that Eastern European women who desire a small family have had little access to or confidence in modern contraceptives. Consequently, by default, abortion has become the major means of limiting fertility in many Eastern European states and the Commonwealth of Independent States (CIS) (formerly the Soviet Union). WHO states that although abortion is legal in these countries, many procedures are carried out under unsanitary conditions or by poorly trained providers. Consequently the complication of unsafe abortions recently accounted for 25–30% of maternal deaths in Russia and an estimated 50% in Albania (Population information Program 2007).

The International Planned Parenthood Federation (IPPF) provided the following information about Eastern Europe:

> According to the 2000 DHS survey in Armenia, around 55% of pregnancies in the three years preceding the survey ended in abortion. According to a UNFPA study in the Khatlon Oblast area of Tajikistan (2000), 64% of respondents of reproductive age had undergone abortions, and 31% had four to five abortions. The high number of abortions is coupled with what is generally acknowledged to be a very poor quality of services, with unsafe abortion making a significant contribution to the high rates of maternal mortality. For example, according to figures published by WHO for 2002, it is estimated that unsafe abortion contributes for approximately 10% of cases of maternal mortality in Kyrgyzstan and 16% in Armenia (WHO 2007). Similarly, in the UNFPA study in Tajikistan 25% of respondents reported having post-abortion complications, which is indicative of poor quality of services. Studies show that poor women, particularly in rural areas, are the most vulnerable (Calverton 2003). Repeat abortions are, to a large extent, due to the very low use of modern contraceptive methods and also reflect the poor quality of post-abortion counselling services. The situation is exacerbated by the high cost of contraception, rendering unsafe abortions a less expensive alternative. Other issues reported to affect the quality of services include the attitudes of gynecologists who view abortion as a good source of income, and outdated Soviet-era guidelines (personal communication April 2007).

This kind of information supports the general points we have made that Eastern European family patterns still differ from Western European patterns and that there is an opportunity to move away from reliance on abortion by improving contraceptive services. We now consider analysis of the situation in larger European countries.

## Austria

The population was estimated at 8.2 million in 2006. Over the period 2000–2005 life expectancy at birth was 79 years. The population is 78% Roman Catholic, 5% Protestant and 17% other religions including Muslim. In the year 2003, the birth rate and the death rate were both nine per thousand. Infant mortality was five per thousand births during 2000–2005. In the 1930s the country had the lowest birth rate in the world (Perner 2007), and in the 1980s the third lowest birth rate after Germany and Italy. In 2005 the average woman had 1.4 children and if trends continue the population will decline to 7.4 million by the year 2050 (Wright 2006: 481). One of the reasons for the decline in birth rate is the reduction in teenage births from 47.0 per thousand in 1960 to only 17.5 per thousand in 1995 (Micklewright and Stewart 1999). The capital city is Vienna with a population of 1.5 million according to the 1991 census (Wright 2006: 532).

At the Hague Forum of 1999, the Austrian government's policy was that government is not called upon to directly influence reproductive behaviour, but that appropriate family policy is to remove, or at least to minimise, those structural obstacles which stand in the way of individuals in their decision to have children. In this respect it outlined a number of measures:

- to improve child care facilities and especially help women with children below school age
- to provide single parents with 18 months off work to have a child; for couples an extra six months between the couple to encourage men to play a more active role
- to carry out job audits on the helpfulness to families and provide government awards to companies which had family friendly policies
- to provide family counselling for those who need it in 305 different centres
- to improve access to family planning to help reduce the abortion rate
- to ensure that family planning was not a population tool but rather a means of extending people's choices
- to make artificial reproduction 'routine' so that more women could benefit.

More recent data reveals that in Austria the higher the qualifications of the woman the lower the percentage of unwanted pregnancies. As of 2007 the country has over 200 publicly supported family planning and partnership counselling centres. As in other countries there was some movement away from oral contraception in the 1970s following scares about its possible adverse effects. Use of the IUD and sterilisation increased. Around 42% of fertile women aged 15–44, however, are still using oral contraception (Perner 2007).

The Austrian abortion law came into force under a Socialist government on 1 January 1975. It was opposed by the Catholic Church which sponsored a 'national petition for the protection of human life'. It was signed by 895,665 people, almost 18% of the electorate. In the introduction to this chapter we have not provided figures of the abortion rate because Austria does not keep records of the number of abortions. The country has allowed in vitro fertilisation since 1992 (Perner 2007).

## Belgium

The population was estimated at 10.4 million in 2006. Over the period 2000–2005 life expectancy at birth was 79 years. The population is 75% Roman Catholic. In the year 2003 the birth rate was 11 per thousand and the death rate ten per thousand, a rate of natural increase of 0.1%. Infant mortality was four per thousand births during 2000–2005. In 2005 the average woman had 1.7 children and if trends continue the population will be 10.2 million by the year 2050 (Wright 2006: 481). The capital city is Brussels with a population of 0.9 million.

Belgium made abortion illegal in 1810 and it was subsequently legalised in 1990. There was a strange case taken to the Bruges Criminal Court when two doctors and a nurse were charged that they did not wait the requisite six days between first appointment and operation when carrying out an abortion on a 14-year-old girl. The girl was 18 at the time of the case, which she had brought herself. A supporter of the doctors said in court that in 25% of cases the six days' waiting time is not adhered to 'due to the woman's urgency and distress' (Genethique 2005).

## Czech Republic

The population was estimated at 10.2 million in 2006. Over the period 2000–2005 life expectancy at birth was 76 years. The population is 40% atheist, 39% Roman Catholic and 5% Protestant (Wright 2006: 564). In the year 2003 the birth rate was nine per thousand and the death rate 11 per thousand, a rate of natural decrease of 0.2%. The infant mortality rate was six per thousand births during 2000–2005. In 2005 the average woman had 1.1 children and if trends continue the population will decline to 8.6 million by the year 2050 (Wright 2006: 482). The capital city is Prague with a population of 1.2 million (1994 estimate).

Czechoslovakia under Alexander Dubček denounced Stalin and abolished censorship, but the brief 'Prague Spring' ended in August 1968 when the Warsaw Pact forces invaded. The Slovaks and Czechs separated on 1 January 1993 and democratic elections were held in 1996.

Abortion was common. In the 1980s there were around 116,000 abortions a year and little use of modern methods of contraception. Alena Kralikova commented: 'Communist leaders sought total control over citizens' (personal communication). Oral contraception was available but fewer than 10% of fertile women used it. The population tended to use the inefficient withdrawal or rhythm methods. Radim Uzel commented: 'The rhythm method was no good for young Czechs. They didn't want to have sex according to a calendar. They wanted to have sex when their parents weren't home' (personal communication). The increase in modern contraception use during the 1980s led to the abortion rate dropping to 58,000. In 2004 the use of oral contraception had increased to two in five fertile women and the number of abortions reduced to 27,574 (Reynolds 2005).

## France

The population was estimated at 60.1 million in 2006. Over the period 2000–2005 its life expectancy at birth was 79 years. The population is 83–88% Roman Catholic, 2% Protestant, 1% Jewish and 5–10% Muslim. In the year 2003 the birth rate was 13 per thousand and the death rate nine per thousand, a rate of natural increase of 0.4%. Infant mortality was five per thousand births during 2000–2005. In 2005 the average woman had 1.9 children and if trends continue the population will be 64.2 million by the year 2050 (Wright 2006: 482). The capital city is Paris with a population of 2.2 million.

French law made abortion illegal in 1810 and the country had a long history of unsafe abortion (Francome 1984a). Tardieu claimed in 1868 that it had increased into a 'veritable industry' and by the end of the century several observers noted the rise in hospital admissions for abortion (Potts et al. 1977: 161). In 1907 a French physician, Tissier, stated that magistrates took a lenient view of abortion and that upper class women had no shame in stating that they had had one (*Lancet* 4 May). In the same report Blondel talked of 'sundry English women, both married and unmarried, who had crossed the channel simply to have an abortion brought on' (pp. 1,257). Other evidence on this issue is provided by a Mrs Burgwin, who visited France around 1913 and told the Birth Rate Commission (1917: 220) that over and over again, doctors had told her that rich English women went to Paris for abortions. One had said, 'We have got 50,000 criminal abortions taking place in Paris in a year and we find numerous English women resort to that city to be relieved of their pregnancy.' This trade continued at least until the 1930s (Ellis 1933).

In the aftermath of the First World War the French government was concerned about low population and in 1920 it introduced a law which even banned contraception. France was thus in the strange position where abortion was provided for foreign women but even birth control was illegal. It seems there were attempts to reduce the number of illegal operations and in 1950 2,885 people were convicted of abortion. In 1969 this number was reduced to 471 and the sentences reduced (*Times* 15 November 1974). One case which brought the issue to prominence was the Bobigny affair, which concerned a girl aged 17 whose pregnancy had been terminated after rape. Her trial took place in November 1972 at Bobigny near Paris. She was acquitted, her mother received a fine and the abortionist a suspended sentence (Francome 1984a: 138).

We have seen in previous works that in both Britain and the USA, activists wishing to change the law had to decide whether to campaign for the right to choose in the early part of pregnancy or whether to settle for more limited change and allow it for rape, incest, fetal abnormality or for social reasons. In France there was an attempt at such a limited bill in 1970 introduced by a Gaullist deputy but, when this failed, the advocates of free abortion demanded repeal in an aggressive campaign. A total of 343 women signed a manifesto published in the left-wing magazine *Le Nouvel Observateur* stating that they had had an abortion and calling for repeal. The list included famous actresses and authors such as Catherine Deneuve, Jeanne Moreau and Simone de Beauvoir and none could be prosecuted because the offences were out of time (*Times* 15 November 1974). Public opinion was in favour of change and the *Catholic Herald* reported that almost 60% of the population was in favour of abortion on demand in the first ten weeks of pregnancy (27 December 1974). Mme Simone Veil, the Minister of Health responsible for the preparation of the bill, claimed that 300,000 French women had abortions each year despite its illegality. This estimate seems high in the light of subsequent experience. The problem of law enforcement was encapsulated by the Minister of the Interior who said that it would have been necessary to send more than 15 million women to prison in the previous 50 years (*Times* 15 November 1974).

We have described events leading to legalisation in more detail elsewhere (Francome 1984a: 138–40). In France, the legalising of abortion on request until the tenth week of pregnancy occurred on 17 Jan 1975. In 1979 the abortion rate was 14.1 per thousand women aged 15–44, then half the rate in the USA. The law was initially on five years' trial. It was a little slow to come into operation but then the numbers of women travelling to England for abortion began to drop rapidly (Francome 1984a: 140).

## Germany

The population was estimated at 82.4 million in 2006. Over the period 2000–2005, life expectancy at birth was 79 years. The population is 34% Protestant, 34% Roman Catholic, 4% Muslim and there are many unaffiliated. In the year 2003 the birth rate was nine per thousand and the death rate ten per thousand, a rate of natural decrease of 0.1%. Infant mortality was five per thousand births during 2000–2005. In 2005 the average woman had 1.3 children and if trends continue the population will decline to 79.1 million by the year 2050 (Wright 2006: 482). The capital city is Berlin with a population of 3.5 million.

The German abortion law was based on the Prussian Penal Code of 1851 which was adopted by the German Reich in 1871 (Kommers 1977). We saw that in April 1971 famous French women publicised their abortions. Inspired by this less than two months later (2 June), 24 well-known actresses, journalists and singers had their photographs on the front page of *Stern* news magazine. All had signed a declaration saying that they had broken German law. These were part of a wider protest where 374 had made the same admission. The youngest was 14 years and the oldest 77. The supporters of liberal abortion used these admissions to argue that the law was unworkable. One of the organisers, Ingrid Huebner, was quoted as saying: 'If all the women who have had an abortion had the courage to take out a summons against themselves the law would be swamped by a flood of 5 million trials.' In theory, under German law, state attorneys have no choice but to prosecute even in cases where a person is self accused. The actress Romy Schneider, despite having a warrant threatening to prosecute her, flew to Bonn to a party given by Chancellor Willy Brandt. This act contravened the terms of the warrant and gave further publicity to the cause (*New York Times* 24 June 1971).

The situation in Germany became acrimonious, with the women's movement arguing that their lives were being controlled by religious doctrines to which they did not subscribe. Churches were daubed with the slogan 'Ban 218', which referred to the relevant clause. On Easter Sunday 1974 the Primate had his service at Munich Cathedral interrupted by a tape-recorded attack on him being released from a confessional booth.

Availability of abortions in other countries led to German women travelling elsewhere. In 1970, 3,621 women travelled to Britain for abortion and the figure quadrupled to 17,531 in 1972. Even more went to Holland and it was estimated that in 1975 a total of 6,000 German women travelled there for abortion. In the same year the number travelling to Britain fell to around 3,400 and by 1984 was only 258 (Francome 1986: 57).

The legalisation in East Germany in 1972 meant that its women had rights to control their fertility not available in the West. Parliament passed a law providing for abortion on request up to 12 weeks' gestation in 1974 but it was referred to the Constitutional Court. One year later this Court overturned the law despite the fact that a poll showed three in five Germans supported it (Francome 1984a: 142). The new law allowed abortion only on such grounds as rape and incest and certain social indicators. This decision led to women travelling to Holland where in 1976 abortions could be obtained for $100 including lunch and coach fare. Access in Germany improved and by 1979 the number of women travelling to Holland had halved from the situation five years earlier (Francome 1984a: 143).

## Greece

The population was estimated at 10.7 million in 2006. Over the period 2000–2005 life expectancy at birth was 78 years. The population is 98% Greek Orthodox and 1.3% Muslim. In the year 2003 both the birth rate and the death rate were 10 per thousand. Infant mortality was 7 per thousand births during 2000–2005. In 2005 the average woman had 1.2 children, half the fertility level of the 1960s, and if trends continue the population will fall to 9.8 million by the year 2050 (Wright 2006: 482). The capital city is Athens with a population of 0.8 million.

We have seen that Western Europe has traditionally had a much higher age of marriage and a much higher percentage of women who never marry than Eastern Europe. Greece shares some of the characteristics of each. The average age of marriage increased from 22.3 years in the 1980s to 25.9 in 1998. The average age of the first child also increased from 23.3 in the 1980s to 28.6 in 1998. Evidence of the continuing respect for marriage in Greece is evidenced by the fact that in 1998 only 3.8% of births occurred outside marriage (Ioannidi-Kapolou 2004):

Traditionally there has always been strict control of women's sexuality, especially in the countryside, with the men of the family responsible for keeping an eye on their daughters and sisters so they do not have sexual relations before or outside marriage (Ioannidi-Kapolou 2004).

Family planning clinics developed in 1980 when the Minister of Health established them in the public sector by law. Ten family planning centres were established. Progress has been slow and Greece has had one of the lowest rates of use of modern contraceptives in Western Europe. It has also concentrated on male methods: in 1997 41% of couples used the condom and a further 31% used withdrawal. This is presumably one of the reasons that the country's abortion rate has been one of the highest in Europe. In the 1970s it was estimated that there were 300,000 illegal abortions carried out each year and women's organisations began to become active on this issue and on contraception.

In 1983 the Greek National Health System was formed; it included information and education on family planning matters amongst its targets. The first published data on induced abortion was in 1965 when a sample of 6,513 married women stated they had had one. There was a ratio of 1:1 abortions to births (Ioannidi-Kapolou 2004). In 1983 the percentage of women who had had an abortion was 36% and rose to 46% by 1997. The percentage of women having had three or more abortions doubled from 9% in 1983 to 18% in 1997. Since Greece legalised abortion in 1986, part of the reason for the increase may well have been that women were more willing to confess to abortion after legalisation. Abortions carried out in government hospitals are free and include the right to three days' leave on full pay. For young women under the age of 18 parental consent is necessary (Ioannidi-Kapolou 2004).

In 2000 a government report estimated that the number of abortions occurring in national hospitals was 100,000–120,000 which, as in 1965, was equal to the number of births. This is an abortion rate over four times as high as, for example, Austria or the Netherlands. This is not the whole picture as many abortions are carried out in gynaecologists' offices and these unregistered abortions are said to number a further 300,000 (Ioannidi-Kapolou 2004). Such figures seem excessive especially as only one in three women aged 35–45 reported they had had an abortion in 2001. This is not much higher than the one in four estimated for Britain. In 2003 over 100,000 prescriptions of emergency contraceptive pills were issued and this may well have led to a decline in the number of abortions.

## Ireland (not including Northern Ireland)

The population was estimated at 4.1 million in 2006. Over the period 2000 to 2005 life expectancy at birth was 78 years. The population is nearly 92% Roman Catholic and 8% other Christian. In the year 2003 the birth rate was 14 per thousand and the death rate eight per thousand, a rate of natural increase of 0.6%. Infant mortality was six per thousand births during 2000–2005. In 2005 the average woman had 1.9 children and if trends continue the population will be 5.0 million by the year 2050 (Wright 2006: 482). The capital city is Dublin with a population of 0.9 million. Ireland's economic position has greatly improved in recent years. In 2004 GNP was USD 34,000 per head, above the figure of USD 33.6 for the UK (Wright 2006: 523–4).

The Irish abortion law is based on the British 1861 Offences Against the Person Act. Public opinion on social issues has historically been very different from the rest of Europe and the USA. For example, a survey in 1973/4 found that 54% of Irish people agreed with the statement 'Divorce should never be allowed'. And seven out of ten stated that sex before marriage is 'always wrong'. It also found that 91% of Catholics went to mass each week. On modern methods of contraception one-third saw them as 'always wrong'. The difference between countries can be seen from a 1980 Gallup poll in Britain, the USA and Ireland which asked a similar question on abortion. In the USA and Ireland the question was 'Do you think abortion should be legal under any circumstances, only under certain circumstances or illegal in all circumstances?' In Britain the phrase 'legal under any circumstances' was substituted by 'legal on demand', but otherwise was identical. The results showed a great difference between Ireland and the other two countries. Whereas four out of five of the Irish thought abortion should be 'illegal in all circumstances', only one in five Americans and one in eight British residents shared that view (Francome 1984: 215). Catholics in Northern Ireland were more liberal than those in the South and 35% would allow abortion in some circumstances.

We have seen that in other countries of the world where abortion is illegal there is a great problem with unsafe operations. However, in Ireland since 1968 women have been able to travel to England. In 1970, 261 Irish women had abortions in Britain. This number increased to 3,603 in 1981 (Francome 1984a: 215). There then followed a steadier increase to 4,200 in 1991 and to 4,900 in 1996; then in 1999 there were 6,200 rising to a high of 6,400 in the year 2000. By this year most other countries had legalised abortion and so their women did not travel to Britain. Consequently more than four out of five (80.5%) of the 9,800 non-resident women having abortions in Britain were from Ireland (both North and South). There has been a move for Irish women to obtain their abortions in Holland where they are cheaper (personal communication).

## Italy

The population was estimated at 58.1 million in 2006. Over the period 2000–2005 its life expectancy at birth was 80 years. The population is mainly Roman Catholic. In the year 2003 the birth rate was nine per thousand and the death rate ten per thousand, a rate of natural decrease of 0.1%. Infant mortality was five per thousand births during 2000–2005. In 2005 the average woman had 1.3 children and if trends continue the population will be 44.9 million by the year 2050 (Wright 2006: 482). The capital city is Rome with a population of 2.7 million (1993).

It seems that abortion was common in Italy even before the First World War: in a large trial in 1904, eight licensed midwives were convicted of what the *British Medical Journal (BMJ)* called 'abortion mongering' (BMJ 28 May 1904). In 1975 the World Health Organization estimated that there were 1.5 million abortions a year, the Italian authorities estimated 800,000 and the women's movement 3 million a year (*Economist* 25 January 1975). A poll in 1976 showed that over three in five (63%) Italians favoured a new law.

The abortion law in Italy was slightly liberalised by a Supreme Court decision of 1976. The law was changed to give women abortion on request on 28 May 1978. The impulse to change the law derived much of its impetus from the developments in France. *The Times* stated: 'France's decision to legalise abortion has left many Italians with a feeling of bitter isolation … all Italy's northern neighbours have now given their women the right to terminate pregnancies under decent and controlled conditions' (6 December 1974).

The campaign in Italy was much different from that in France and Britain where the pro-choice organisations tried to keep a more respectable image and argued, for example, that abortion would protect the family. In contrast Italian feminist groups began confrontational tactics. The Centro Informazione Sterilizzione e Aborto (CISA) aimed to help women directly and make the country face up to the issue. It introduced suction abortion to Italy and accompanied women to cheap practitioners or, if their pregnancy had passed three months, to London. It was headed by Adele Faccio a 55-year-old single woman who bore a son at the age of 36. She was speaking in Paris when she learned she was to be arrested and gained maximum publicity by announcing she would give herself up at a large abortion rally in Rome. She returned to Italy with the help of borrowed documents and a wig to force the arrest to take place in front of the press, television and hundreds of supporters. *The Times* commented: 'The episode has the desired effect of turning Adele Faccio into a heroine and martyr and making the embarrassed carabinieri officer appear the stooge of an obtuse regime bent on imposing its crude fascist laws' (15 April 1976).

One of the crucial issues of the debate was the relationship between Church and State. This problem had become accentuated with the 'Seveso' case when an explosion led to women being exposed to a chemical known to cause fetal malformation. The Christian Democrats allowed 38 women to have abortions, a decision that caused a rift with the Vatican (*Catholic Herald* 20 August 1976; *Universe* 7 July 1978).

In 1979, the first full year after the act, 188,000 legal abortions occurred at the expense of the state. This is below the level of unsafe abortions estimated but was three times the number of abortions carried out by the British health service in the same year.

The country had to decide whether to overthrow the law in a referendum. The Catholic Church played an active role and the *Observer* commented: 'The Pope has virtually entered the hustings' (3 May 1981). The people defeated the 'pro-life' amendments with 67.9% of people opposed to it. Even before the voting, Joan Lewis, in Rome for the *Catholic Herald*, predicted the final result:

> There is a silent majority in this predominantly Catholic country which admits that abortion is here to stay, however heart rending and agonizing the problem. The more vocal of this majority argue that it would be better to search deeper and find the causes of this 'social plague' as they call it. They say that abrogating the current law would not eliminate abortions and indeed, could encourage clandestine abortions, which have a high mortality rate. (Francome 1984a: 146)

Both the Italian abortion rate and the birth rate have declined in recent years, which indicates that contraceptive methods have become more efficient.

## The Netherlands

The population was estimated at 16.5 million in 2006. Over the period 2000–2005 life expectancy at birth was 78 years. The population is 31% Roman Catholic, 21% Protestant, 40% unaffiliated and 3% Muslim. In the year 2003 the birth rate was 12 per thousand and the death rate nine per thousand, a rate of natural increase of 0.3%. Infant mortality was five per thousand births during 2000–2005. In 2005 the average woman had 1.7 children and if trends continue the population will be 17 million by the year 2050 (Wright 2006: 483). The capital city is Amsterdam with a population of 0.7 million.

The greatest difference between developments in Holland and those in other countries is that the big increase in quasi-legal abortion preceded any change in the law. A Dutch abortion law of 1836 had proved to be ineffective as it had been necessary to prove that the fetus was alive at the time of the operation. In 1911 the law was changed so that abortion was also considered to be a crime against public morality (Ketting and Schnabel 1980). From this time onwards there were abortions only on 'medical grounds' and in the 1950s an estimated 10,000–15,000 illegal abortions a year (Treffers 1965: 58).

Although the Dutch were amongst the first pioneers of contraception in the nineteenth century, it appears that progress was slow. One strong belief reported was that a birth control mentality was a major cause of induced abortion and this was to be discouraged. However, with the introduction of oral contraception in 1964 it became accepted that contraception could prevent abortion, and in a small country such as Holland the use of oral contraception spread rapidly. In 1969 the ban on birth control advertising was lifted and by 1971 the cost of female-orientated methods was covered by the country's public health insurance and thus free of charge. By 1977, 41% of Dutch women aged 15–44 were taking oral contraception – by far the highest usage in the world. This change in contraception practice had led to different attitudes about abortion. In cases where contraception failed, physicians felt responsible and women began to believe in the right to control their own fertility.

In 1966 an eminent Dutch law professor, Ch J Enschede, concluded that the concept of what was 'medical' had become much broader amongst physicians and that this should apply to abortion as well. He concluded that doctors were well within their rights under the law if they carried out abortions on a wide variety of social grounds, such as if the woman were single or had completed her family. The statement seems to have taken the medical profession by surprise. However, in the following year it was approved in parliament by the secretary of justice, and it became accepted that any abortion carried out in proper conditions by a doctor was legal (de Bruijn 1979: 192; Ketting and Schnabel 1980). In the late 1960s there was, however, a shortage of capacity and in 1970, 816 Dutch women had abortions in Britain. However, the setting up of specialist clinics from 1971 avoided the need for women to travel and in 1973 only 101 Dutch women had abortions in England (Francome 1984a: 136). Indeed, foreign women began to travel to Holland for abortions. Although the abortion rate for resident women was low – only around 5.2 abortions per thousand women aged 15–45 years, the influx of foreigners was estimated by Stimezo – the Dutch National Abortion Federation – to be as high as 61,000 from Germany, 12,000 from Belgium and 9,000 from France in 1975 (Ketting and Schnabel 1980).

Despite the low abortion rate and presence of legal abortion, introducing a bill to regularise the situation was controversial. As we have documented more fully elsewhere, there were a total of eight bills in 11 years, before in 1981 a bill allowed abortion on request up to 20 weeks' gestation in specially licensed clinics but required a five-day 'meditation' period between the request and the operation (Francome 1984a: 137).

## Norway

The population was estimated at 4.6 million in 2006. Over the period 2000–2005 life expectancy at birth was 79 years. The population is 86% Evangelical Lutheran, 3% other Protestant, 1% Roman Catholic and 10% no religion. In the year 2003 the birth rate was 12 per thousand and the death rate 10 per thousand, a rate of natural increase of 0.2%. In 2005 the average woman had 1.8 children and if trends continue the population will be 4.9 million by the year 2050 (Wright 2006: 482). The rate of maternal mortality fell from around 500 deaths per 100,000 births in 1880 to 10 per 100,000 in 1979 and 4.6 per 100,000 in the 1990s, one of the lowest rates in the world. The capital city is Oslo with a population of 483,000 (Wright 2006: 644)

The first clinic offering advice related to sexuality and childbearing was opened in Oslo and others followed. Contraceptive advice was limited at first, but it gradually expanded and by the 1960s when modern contraceptives became available there was already a tradition of family planning. In 1999 the government decided to provide free condoms to all young people under the age of 20. These were introduced to help reduce the abortion rate and as a strategy to reduce the incidence of HIV and sexually transmitted infections. In 2002 parliament decided that women under the age of 20 were to receive free contraceptive pills (Austveg and Sundby 2005).

The Norwegian abortion law of 1687 did not distinguish between abortion and infanticide and punished them both with the death penalty. Capital punishment was replaced by hard labour and prison in 1842. The Penal Code of 1902, which remained in place until 1964, allowed abortions if they were justified by a doctor. The number of illegal abortions resulting in maternal deaths rose steadily at the beginning of the twentieth century and then doubled during the decade 1920–1930. During the period 1930–1940 these deaths rose only slightly but were high during the war years of 1940 to 1945, although local observers say some of this might be attributable to better reporting. (Austveg and Sundby 2005: 25). In post-war years illegal abortion deaths began to fall rapidly until they were much lower by the early 1950s (Austveg and Sundby 2005). In 1964 a law came into force requiring hospital medical committees to decide all individual cases. A study in 1973 documented social and geographical differences in the decision of doctors and medical committees as to whether legal abortion should be provided. The modern law came into operation in 1979 and allows 'abortion on demand' in the first 12 weeks of pregnancy and by a decision of a medical committee over 12 weeks (Austveg and Sundby 2005: 25).

When abortion was legalised some felt that the rate would rise, but that did not occur. In 1980 the abortion rate was 16.3 per thousand aged 15–45. In 2002 the abortion rate for women aged 15–49 (a slightly different age range) was only 12.6 and the overall trend has been downwards (Francome 1984a: 129). Abortion rates amongst adolescents (under 20) fell from 21.0 per thousand in 1982 to 16.9 in 2002. This reduction is despite the fact that the reported age of first intercourse has reduced by one year over the past ten years and is presently 16.7 years of age. Norway was one of the pioneers in the introduction of in vitro fertilisation treatment in public hospitals.

## Poland

The population was estimated at 38.5 million in 2006. Over the period 2000–2005 life expectancy at birth was 74 years. The population is 95% Roman Catholic (about 75% practising) (Wright 2006: 652). In 1920 the birth rate was 37.6 per thousand and declined to 22.3 in 1960 (Francome 1984a: 130). In the year 2003 the birth rate was 11 per thousand, which is less than a third of its 1920 level. The death rate was ten per thousand which gives a rate of natural increase of 0.1%. Infant mortality was nine per thousand births during 2000–2005. In 2005 the average woman had 1.3 children and if trends continue the population will decline to 33 million by the year 2050 (Wright 2006: 483). The capital city is Warsaw with a population of 1.6 million (1994 estimate).

A 1932 law allowed abortion for the sake of the woman's health and for rape and incest. Abortion was legalised on request in 1955 and this led to Swedish women travelling to Poland for terminations. In 1965 the New York Times (14 February) reported that Swedish law stated that it was illegal to do abroad what it was illegal to do in Sweden and so 20 women were threatened with prosecution. This resulted in great opposition and led to a revision of the Swedish law. In the year 1978 Poland had 145,600 abortions recorded, a rate of 18.3 per thousand women aged 15–44, although this figure is recognised as being incomplete (Francome 1984a: 129). Maria told us of her experience:

> In 1987 I was just splitting up from my husband of sixteen years. We had never used contraception and only had one child. When we broke up I had a brief affair with a policeman. He was very high up not one who was on the streets. He was married and I was very surprised when I became pregnant. I did not feel I had any choice but to have an abortion. He paid for me to go to a private clinic and the abortion was very painful. The cost was equal to a month's pay (interview 3 April 2007).

Since the country has been independent of Communist rule the law has been controversial. First, abortion was restricted in 1993, and there was some concern about illegal abortion which was a factor in the law's being legalised on wider grounds in October 1996. It figured heavily in the election of the following year which led to it being restricted once again. The current law allows abortion for the woman's health or life, for fetal abnormality or for such crimes as rape or incest. There is further pressure from the Right to make abortion illegal even for rape. The prime minister, Jaroslaw Kaczynski, rejected this call from the League of Polish Families to provide the 'right to life from the moment of conception'. He was quoted as saying: 'Can a sovereign and democratic state oblige a woman who has been raped to have a baby. In my opinion it cannot.' Such a restriction would not have had the support of public opinion as only one in five (20%) supported stricter abortion laws (Easton 2007).

It is estimated that there are 200,000 illegal abortions a year and the illegal sector is said to be 'thriving' (Moore 2003). Many women also travel to the Czech Republic where abortion is legal and the Swedes have stated that they should help Polish women who want abortions to repay the favour for earlier periods where Poland provided abortion for Swedish women as we have discussed (Francome 2004a). However, Polish women have died because of the presence of unsafe abortions. For example, in March 2005 Karina Kozak underwent an illegal abortion in the private apartment of a gynaecologist. After the procedure she haemorrhaged and was taken by ambulance to a hospital where she died. Less than two months later a 25-year-old pregnant woman became ill during pregnancy and the medical profession failed to carry out the appropriate procedure. The doctor said he had planned to perform an endoscopy, which carries the risk of miscarriage, but decided against it: 'My conscience won't let me do it.' The woman died and Professor Rydzewska said that if the endoscopy had been performed it would have identified the source of infection and the problem would have been solved (Nowicka 2005: 162). The reintroduction of illegal abortion to Poland and problems with care for the health of the pregnant woman is creating a difficult situation.

In 2003 Wanda Nowicka, the president of the Polish Federation for Women and Family Planning, saw the fruits of her invitation to the Dutch group 'Women on Waves' as they visited the country. The group moored their boat in Wladyslawowo but planned to go to international waters in order to provide women who were up to six weeks pregnant with RU 486. Its leader, Dr Rebecca Gomperts, commented:

What I can I tell you is that we've had more than 200 telephone calls from the public. Women are desperate here. You cannot imagine how a woman feels when she has an unwanted pregnancy. She doesn't want a child and she feels so lonely. It is very sad and moving when you talk to these women (Moore 2003).

Other women said that the boat had opened discussion. For example, 20-year-old Olga described her experience a year earlier. She was about to take exams and commented:

> I was not ready to have a baby. I answered an ad in a newspaper and found a doctor. I had to pay a lot of money for the abortion. I think it is a good idea that Women on Waves came to Poland. More women feel confident about discussing abortion now (Moore 2003).

A case to the European Court has thrown the law in Poland into some disarray. In February 2000 Alicja Tysiac became pregnant with her third child. She went to see three specialists who all said that continuing the pregnancy was likely to cause deterioration in her vision. However, as they felt the potential deterioration was not certain they refused to authorise abortion. She continued with the pregnancy and her eyesight deteriorated to such a degree that she could only see up to five feet away. She took the Polish government to the European Court of Human Rights and in March 2007 she was awarded 25,000 euros compensation. At the press conference following the decision she commented:

> Every woman should decide herself whether she wants to have the baby or not and the government should not mix into that at all … In Poland there is no work, people have nowhere to live and it is hard to see your own child hungry or to deny it things.

In addition to these comments Wanda Nowicka alleged: 'Thousands of women are denied abortions that they are legally entitled to in Poland every year.' The government had three months to appeal the decision but it is likely to have ramifications; the Irish government is also concerned as it has a similar case due to come before the court (Easton 2007; Hennesy and Smyth 2007).

In March 2007 the Polish prime minister rebuked his deputy over the issues of gays and abortion. Roman Giertych of the far-right League of Polish Families had called on the EU to stop propaganda in favour of homosexuality and support for abortion rights. The European parliament was critical of the 'rise in racist, xenophobic, anti-Semitic and homophobic intolerance'.

We saw in the Introduction that a Polish clinic providing in vitro fertilisation was ordered to close in 2007 because it was said to breach the abortion law. One in six Polish couples are estimated to suffer from infertility problems (Perlez 2007).

## Portugal

The population was estimated at 10.6 million in 2006. Over the period 2000–2005 life expectancy at birth was 77 years. The population is 94% Roman Catholic, but only one-third are regular churchgoers. In the year 2003 the birth rate was 12 per thousand and the death rate 10 per thousand, a rate of natural decrease of 0.2%. Infant mortality was six per thousand births during 2000–2005. In 2005 the average woman had 1.4 children and if trends continue the population will reduce to 9 million by the year 2050 (Wright 2006: 483). The capital city is Lisbon with a population of 0.7 million (1991 census).

The inauguration of democracy in 1974 led to women's rights becoming a crucial issue. The new constitution introduced in 1975 recognised the right to a new 'conscious parenthood', but abortion remained a crime. In 1976 the Family Planning Association was founded and the abortion issue was brought to prominence by a film called, ironically, *Abortion is not a Crime*. It showed an abortion by use of a Karman's canula and bicycle pump, and made it reasonably easy to see how to carry one out. The programme also included a discussion in a dimly lit room with a group of women who explained they had had abortions. The journalist who wrote the script, Mario Palla, was charged in 1979 with 'assault on public morals' and incitement to crime. Palla's position on the issue was clear: 'To legalize abortion is a real concrete way to make women more free. People who are against the liberalization of women are against abortion' (Francome 1984a: 213).

A bill was passed in 1984 which allowed abortion in the first 12 weeks of pregnancy for the woman's health and for rape until 16 weeks. There was pressure to further change the law and in 1998 a referendum asked the following question: 'Do you agree with decriminalisation of abortion when requested on women's demand up to 10 weeks of pregnancy and performed in an authorised clinic?' The turnout was low at only 32%. A bare 50.1% voted 'No'. On 13 July it was announced that the law in Portugal was coming into effect on 15 July. It legalises abortion on request up to ten weeks of pregnancy after a mandatory three-day waiting period (Associated Press 2007). This, of course, did not end abortion and in the year 2007 around 40,000 abortions were estimated to have occurred each year. Richer women could go to Spain and clinics were built just over the border in relatively easy reach of Portuguese women. Others were carried out locally by *partieras* – 'capable women'. These were part of a long tradition: as long ago as 1979 one of the activists, Madelena Barbosa, was quoted as saying: 'Some of the midwives are really quite good, they use proper medical instruments and operate in sterile conditions' (Francome 1984a: 214). There were several high profile prosecutions on the grounds of illegal abortion. One such was of JA Pinto, a social worker, who said that every week he encountered women who wanted illegal abortions. Pinto was freed on appeal but others were sent to prison. The new referendum took place on 11 February 2007 and had the support of the Socialist prime minister who was quoted as saying: 'We have to end this plight of backstreet abortions. It makes Portugal a backward place' (Catalinotti 2007). In the referendum 60% of the respondents were in support of a new law. However, although the turnout was increased to 44%, it did not reach the 50% required for the decisions to be mandatory.

## Romania

The population was estimated at 22.3 million in 2006. Over the period 2000–2005 life expectancy at birth was 71 years. The population is 87% Eastern Orthodox, 6% Roman Catholic and 7% Protestant. In the year 2003 the birth rate was 11 per thousand and the death rate 12 per thousand, a rate of natural decrease of 0.1%. Infant mortality was 18 per thousand births during 2000–2005. In 2005 the average woman had 1.3 children and if trends continue the population will be 18.1 million by the year 2050 (Wright 2006: 483). The capital city is Bucharest with a population of 2.1 million (1993 estimate). Contraceptive use increased from over half (57%) of married and cohabiting women in 1990 to two-thirds (65%) in the year 2000. However, only one in three (31%) women were using modern methods of contraception (UN 2004: 57).

Abortion was first legalised in September 1957 following legal changes in the Soviet Union. Romania provides a good example of what can happen to women's health if abortion is prohibited. In 1966 the government, concerned about declining fertility and population growth placed stringent restrictions on the liberal Abortion Act. Decree 770 stated that abortion would be allowed only under the following conditions:

- they had given birth to and raised four or more children, or were over 40 years of age
- they suffered from or had a spouse who suffered from a severe hereditary disease which might be transmitted
- they had severe physical, psychological or sensory disabilities that would prevent them from caring for the newborn
- their life was threatened or the pregnancy was the result of rape or incest.

Until this time the number of deaths from abortion had been falling. Deaths halved from 130 in 1961 to 64 in 1965. However, they then almost tripled to 170 in 1967 and increased by over five times to 364 in 1971. This rise in abortion deaths was clearly related to the growth in unsafe operations after the criminalisation of abortion. Over the same period the birth rate shows the effect of the law. It was 17.5 per thousand population in 1961 and steadily fell together with the abortion deaths to 14.6 per thousand in 1965. It then almost doubled to 27.4 in 1967. However, as the number of illegal operations began to rise, the birth rate steadily fell and by 1971 it was 19.5 per thousand which is down by almost a third from the peak (Francome 1976: 392).

The restrictive abortion law in Romania lasted for 24 years until December 1989 when the dictator Nicolae Ceausescu was executed and the new government made abortion legal on request (Johnson et al. 2004: 184). Observers commented:

> Although abortion became much safer, quality of care was severely limited by the heavy demand for services. In the early 1990s the disastrous effects of Ceausescu's extreme pro-natalist anti family planning policies on women's sexual and reproductive lives were documented (Johnson et al. 2004: 184).

After the law changed, deaths from abortion reduced. In 1989 maternal mortality was 170 deaths per 100,000 live births and 87% of all maternal deaths were abortion related. The rate more than halved to 84 per 100,000 in 1990 and then to 53 per 100,000 in 1993. This decline was due almost entirely to the decrease in abortion-related mortality from 148 per 100,000 live births in 1989 to under a quarter – 34 per 100,000 – in 1993. By 2002, abortion-related mortality was down to nine per 100,000 (Johnson 2004: 186). The exceptionally low rates of contraception led to the country having possibly the highest abortion rate in the world from 1990 to 1992. Teams assessing abortion interviewed a woman in the Roma community who freely admitted performing 24 abortions on herself with a pen and having no complications (Johnson 2004: 189). The rate was 182 abortions per thousand women of reproductive age which is around 30 times the rate of some other Western countries such as Germany, Holland and Belgium. There were three abortions for every live birth.

The end of the Ceausescu regime led the way for the World Bank to give financial assistance to reproductive health and Romania is now considered to be one of the success stories of the countries that were part of the USSR. In Romania it was general practitioners rather than gynaecologists who provided the contraceptive counselling and by the end of 2003, 2,300 of approximately 15,000 family doctors had been trained together with 1,750 nurses (Johnson 2004). By 2004 there were around 250 clinics and the Ministry of Health had also implemented a programme to provide free contraceptives to poor and disadvantaged women. In 2002 the rate was 32 abortions per thousand women of reproductive health, which is below a fifth its rate in 1990 to 1992, but is still relatively high; it does seem to indicate that improvements in contraceptive services could lead to further reductions. It seems that the services are intimidating to teenagers and that there are problems of access in rural areas. In addition, whereas doctors are trained in providing oral contraception, women wanting an intra-uterine device (IUD) can receive it only from a gynaecologist. There are few doctors trained in providing vasectomies. The authorities are attempting to improve matters. The price of abortions had remained nominal for around ten years at $2, although women often gave the practitioner a gift of money or a present on top of this figure. In 2004 the official price was doubled by the Ministry of Health in conjunction with offering free contraceptives to those having abortions (Johnson et al. 2004: 190). This change, together with other developments, is likely to further reduce the abortion rate.

## Russian Federation

The population was estimated at 142.9 million in 2006. Over the period 2000–2005 life expectancy at birth was 65 years. The population is Russian Orthodox with Muslims predominating in some areas, although the dominant ideology was atheism during the Communist years. In the year 2003 the birth rate was 10 per thousand and the death rate 14 per thousand, a rate of natural decrease of 0.4%. Infant mortality was 17 per thousand births during 2000–2005. In 2005 the average woman had 1.4 children and if trends continue the population will decline by 31 million to 111.8 million by the year 2050 (Wright 2006: 483). The capital, Moscow, has a population of 8.7 million. St Petersburg has a population of 4.8 million (1995 data) (Wright 2006: 658).

It was in the Soviet Union that abortion was first legalised in modern times, and the developments there strongly affected the debate in Britain and the USA. As early as 1914 the most eminent society of physicians had called for all laws to be removed. In 1920 the Soviet government, faced with a birth rate of about 40 per thousand and a high number of unsafe abortions passed a law legalising the operation (Francome 1984a). It provided that the operation would be performed free of charge in hospitals, although a shortage of resources meant that the law could not be implemented.

The Soviet law had two main effects on the debate elsewhere. First, it was a prime example to show that change was possible, and radical groups were able to point to it as an example of what could be accomplished. Second, and this was probably more important, it revised the estimates of the safety of the operation. Until that time it had been believed that abortion was an unsafe operation. The Soviet authorities drew comparisons with Germany where in 1924 4% of abortions were estimated to have resulted in death. In contrast, the Moscow death rate was less than one-tenth of 1% (*New Generation* September 1926). The Soviets publicised their results and in 1929 sent a delegate to the first congress of the World League for Sexual Reform in London. The figures suggested that abortion mortality and morbidity in the country had decreased 'almost to vanishing point'. British doctors took a great interest and on a number of occasions visited the country to observe the procedures. One such doctor was L Haden Guest, who reported in the *Lancet* (5 December 1931) that in a Russian series of 40,000 abortions there were only two deaths. The US-based Dr FJ Taussig paid a visit to the Soviet Union in 1930 and devoted a whole chapter of his influential book to legal abortion in the country (Francome 1984a: 63; Taussig 1936).

In 1936 the Soviet Union repealed its law. The *New York Times* reported strong opposition from women who felt they would be condemned to being childbearing machines, commenting that the abortion law had not prevented the creation of happy, devoted and even conventional families. It argued that the change in the law was 'the first step toward pitting the Soviet Union squarely into a population race with Germany and Italy' (7 March 1937). The change in the law was accompanied by promises of large premiums for every child after the seventh and there was also a crackdown on illegal abortion. In one case 18 women were sentenced to between one and ten years in prison. The restricted Soviet law continued to allow abortion if pregnancy threatened the woman's health or if there was a likelihood of inherited disease (Francome 1984a: 63). The programme was initially successful and official estimates told of a tripling of the birth rate in Moscow in the first year (Francome 1984a: 64).

The Soviet Union legalised abortion again in 1956 and the law became fully operational in 1958. It was legal on request until 12 weeks' gestation and up to 20 weeks on a variety of social grounds. Russia had a very high rate of abortions: in 1959 it was recorded at 165 per thousand women in the fertile age group. In 1960 it fell substantially to 110 and fluctuated around this figure for 20 years and was 123 in 1980 (Johnston 2007a). It then fell over the next ten years until it was 67 in 1990. In 1992 the government began to subsidise contraception and during the 1990s the abortion rate fell further to 55 per thousand in 2000 and 45 in 2004. During the period 1988–2001 the percentage of women using modern contraception increased by 74% while the number of abortions decreased by 61% (Deschner and Cohen 2003; Johnston 2007a).

There are signs that with the resurgence of the Russian Orthodox Church and concerns with declining population there have been some attempts to reduce the number of abortions by legal means; in 2003 the government restricted the social grounds for abortion after 12 weeks' gestation. The right to choose remained in the first 12 weeks. This was a relatively small change but nevertheless was opposed by Dr Yuri Bloshansky, who had been Moscow's chief gynaecologist for over 40 years. He said, 'I remember vividly the women dying, forced to go anywhere, going to swindlers operating in septic conditions' (Myers 2003).

## Spain

The population was estimated at 40.4 million in 2006. Over the period 2000–2005 life expectancy at birth was 79 years. The population is 94% Roman Catholic, but local observers comment that church attendance is dwindling and fewer than 20% go to mass regularly (Adler 2004; da Cunha e Tavora 2007). In the year 2003 the birth rate was ten per thousand and the death rate nine per thousand, a rate of natural increase of 0.1%. Infant mortality was five per thousand births during 2000–2005. In 2005 the average woman had 1.3 children and if trends continue the population will decline by 3 million to 37.3 million by the year 2050 (Wright 2006: 483). However, the number of births has increased from just under 1.1 per woman in 2000 (Westen 2006a). The capital city is Madrid with a population of 3 million. Contraceptive use increased from seven in ten (70%) married and cohabiting women in 1990 to nine in ten (92%) in the year 2000 and of these over four out of five (82%) used modern methods of contraception (UN 2004: 57).

One of the first liberalisations of the abortion law in Western Europe was in Catalonia which, in 1936, allowed abortion for fetal deformity, rape or 'sentimental' reasons in the first three months (Aderson 1980). The movement to the Right under the rule of General Franco in the late thirties led to abortion, birth control and divorce being made illegal. After he died a new constitution was set up which paved the way for birth control to be legalised in 1978 and divorce in 1981. In 1974 the Spanish Council of Scientific Investigations came to the conclusion that the abortion law was inadequate and should be revised. The setting up of a democratic system led to the parties dividing, with the left-wing groups being more in favour than the right-wing groups (Aderson 1980). The major pressure for change came from the women's movement. There have been many trials and in 1975 there were 151, for example, and *Spare Rib* (December 1979) reported that a woman had received ten years' imprisonment. It was, however, the twice- suspended trial of eleven women in Bilbao which most galvanised opinion. Nine of the women had undergone abortions and almost all of them already had several children. The tenth person was the abortionist and the eleventh her daughter who had helped. The trial began in October 1979. As in France and Italy one of the most effective protests was from well-known women who stated they had had abortions. In Spain 4,300 women including a respected dramatic actress, the Eurovision Song Contest winner, and a former Miss Spain signed a statement which in part pointed out 'Spanish justice is condemning women because they do not have the £250 which it costs to go to England for an abortion' (*Guardian* 25 October 1979). This protest brought great publicity to the trial and when it concluded in March 1982 ten of the 11 women were cleared. The abortionist, Julia Garcia, was found guilty but was recommended for an immediate pardon.

One estimate in the late 1970s was that overall there were 300,000 abortions each year in Spain. Many women began to seek legal terminations in Britain. The first record of Spanish terminations in the UK was in 1972 when 730 were performed. The number rose to 2,900 in 1974 and it had reached 14,100 by 1978 and 22,000 by 1983. In January 1983 the newly elected Socialist government published plans to liberalise the law in cases of rape, fetal deformity and risk to the life of the woman (*Daily Telegraph* 28 January 1983). The Spanish law was changed in 1985. It was article 417 of the Penal Code of the Organic Law No. 9 1985. It allowed abortion in the following cases:

- To avoid physical or mental harm to the mother. Two doctors must give their consent.
- Rape or incest was declared to the police. This was only in the first 12 weeks.
- The fetus was severely physically or mentally handicapped (allowed up to 22 weeks).

If these conditions were met, the social security would pay 75% of the costs (Fuchs 2005). An estimate from 2003 was that over 97% of the abortions occurred under the first condition, 2.5% under the second condition and 0.1% were because of rape (*Life Site News* 2003). With the change in the law the number of women travelling abroad began to reduce. By the year 2000 only 32 residents of Spain had abortions in Britain (Francome 2004a: 41). This might seem a little surprising as the law does not seem particularly liberal. The BBC correspondent in Spain commented: 'The way Spanish women get around the situation is to sign a piece of paper testifying that if they do not abort, they will suffer psychologically' (Adler 2004). In fact, the interpretation of the law was such that some British women went to Spain for later abortions which would have been illegal in Britain.

The number of abortions in Spain increased from 49,000 in 1995 to 85,000 in 2004. This rise may have been in part due to a decline in illegal abortion, but Pilar Triguero of CEAPA, a national federation of 12,500 parent–teacher associations asserted:

We have to get rid of the taboos about sex education. The state-funded schools tiptoe around the subject and they do not have an established curriculum. What is taught depends on the discretion of each teacher (Fuchs 2005).

A different reason was suggested by Margarita Delgado, a demographer, who said that the many women waited for a permanent job until they decided to start a family. Spanish businesses worked late hours which made it difficult for women to juggle jobs and children. She added that state support for families in Spain was one of the lowest in the European Union (Fuchs 2005).

There is a movement towards legal abortion on request in the first 12 weeks of pregnancy. An early decision on this has been postponed (Adler 2004).

## Sweden

The population was estimated at 9.0 million in 2006. Over the period 2000–2005 life expectancy at birth was 80 years. The population is 87% Lutheran. In the year 2003 the birth rate was 11 per thousand and the death rate 10 per thousand, a rate of natural increase of 0.1%. Infant mortality was three per thousand births during 2000–2005. In 2005 the average woman had 1.7 children and if trends continue the population will be 8.7 million by the year 2050 (Wright 2006: 483). The capital city is Stockholm with a population of 0.7 million.

In the seventeenth century Sweden had made abortion punishable by death. In 1864 it reduced the punishment to six years in prison (Linner 1968). Sweden liberalised its law in 1921 but the restrictions meant that illegal abortion still continued; during the 1930s they caused around 70 deaths each year. A Royal Commission was set up in 1934 and resulting legislation went into operation on 1 January 1939. It allowed abortion if childbirth would entail serious danger to the life or health of the woman, of if she were pregnant from rape or incest or under 15 years of age. It also allowed abortion in cases where the woman was legally insane or if serious physical or mental handicap might result (Linner 1968: 76). In 1946 a further indication was added. This was to allow abortion if there were reasons to assume that childbirth and care would seriously undermine the woman's physical and psychological strength with reference to her living conditions and other special circumstances. In 1956 Sweden made sex education compulsory. The drug thalidomide gave prominence to the abortion issue. First marketed for morning sickness in 1957, it was by 1962 known to be responsible for deformed children. The drug was not accepted in the USA but a US journalist, Sherri Finkbine, had been prescribed the drug in England; when she could not get a legal abortion in the USA, and amongst great publicity, she flew to Sweden for an abortion.

Although Swedish law was more liberal than others it was still very bureaucratic. In the period 1963–1964 the patients at one hospital had an average of 26 days investigation and spent an average ten days in hospital (Potts et al. 2007). Abortion was more easily available in Sweden and in the winter of 1964–1965, 20 women were threatened with prosecution. Swedish law stated that it was illegal to do abroad what it was illegal to do in Sweden (*New York Times* 14 February 1965). The predictable furore led to the prosecution being dropped and an eight-member commission to review the law. This recommended in 1971 that abortion should be removed from the Penal Code, although abortions by lay persons should be illegal. In 1973 the law in Sweden was changed to allow abortion on request in the first 18 weeks of pregnancy. Between 12 and 18 weeks there must, however, be a discussion with a social worker (Francome 1984a: 132–4). In the 1990s the Swedish birth rate was higher than virtually all the countries in Western Europe. This has been linked to the introduction of 15-month parental leave and a doubling in the number of day centres. One observer suggested that if other countries wished to increase their birth rate they should provide parents with the time and resources to raise their children well (Arthur 1999). The Swedish abortion rate in the period 1998–2004 was just over 20 per thousand women aged 15–44, which we have seen is twice as high as countries such as Holland or Switzerland (Johnston 2005).

The Swedish law gave indigenous women the right to choose and in 2005 a government-commissioned report said the residential requirement should be waived. This was followed by an announcement on 16 January 2007. It was quickly noticed by the Poles who suggested that Polish women would be able to get safe legal abortions in the country (Szczech 2007).

## Ukraine

The population was estimated at 46.7 million in 2006. Over the period 2000–2005 life expectancy at birth was 66 years. This is a reduction from 70.5 in 1990 and 68.1 in 1999 (Hovorun and Vornyk 2003). In 2005 the average woman had 1.1 children and if trends continue the population will be reduced to 26.4 million by the year 2050 (Wright 2006: 483). In the year 2003 the birth rate was 10 per thousand and the death rate 16 per thousand, a rate of natural decrease of 0.6%. Infant mortality was 16 per thousand births during 2000–2005. The capital city is Kiev with a population of 2.6 million (1995 estimate). The religious background is around 75% Eastern Orthodox, 13.5% Roman Catholic, 2.3% Jewish and 8% Baptist and other Christian groups (Hovorun and Vornyk 2003). The country achieved its independence in 1991 but had an extreme financial crisis in 1991/2. Inflation rose from 4% in 1990 to 85% in 1991 (UN 1995). Some of the financial problems of the society are due to the nuclear accident in Chernobyl.

Like the other countries of the former USSR, the country has had a tradition of relatively low contraception and high abortion rates. In Kiev for example in 1982, amongst sexually active women aged 19 and under, 78% were using no contraceptives, 10% used abortion, 8% used contraception and 4% both contraception and abortion. In 1974 the government effectively blocked access to the contraceptive pill (Hovorun and Vornyk 2003). In 1982 there were 1.6 million pregnancies and 700,000 abortions (UN 1995).

In recent years contraception has improved but still estimates suggest that there are 1.2 abortions per women. The government wishes to reduce the rate; consequently in January 2003 a new policy on the family was introduced. This made the legal rights of couples cohabiting much the same as of those who were married. It aimed to increase financial support for women in the hope that this would reduce the number of abortions occurring for financial reasons.

## United Kingdom

Great Britain consists of England, Scotland and Wales. The addition of Northern Ireland is called the UK. The population was estimated at 60.6 million in 2006. Over the period 2000 to 2005 life expectancy at birth was 78 years. The population is 66% Anglican and Roman Catholic; other Christian groups make up about 3%. There are about 2.4% Muslims, nearly 1% of both Sikhs and Hindus and 0.6% Jews. In the year 2003 the birth rate was 11 per thousand and the death rate 10 per thousand, a rate of natural increase of

0.1%. Infant mortality was five per thousand births during 2000–2005. In 2005 the average woman had 1.7 children and if trends continue the population will be 66.2 million by the year 2050 (Wright 2006: 483). The capital city is London with a population of 7 million (1994 estimate).

The early debate on contraception was rooted in the ideas of Thomas Malthus and his theory that there was a natural tendency for population size to outstrip food supply. He proposed that poor people should engage in self-restraint in order to restrict their family size. The neo-Malthusian movement altered his doctrine by suggesting people should use contraception rather than restraint. Two of its members published a booklet about contraception called The *Fruits of Philosophy*, and were brought to trial. The Solicitor General argued that the real aim of the book was 'to suggest to people that they might enjoy the pleasures of sexual intercourse with or without marriage and yet avoid offspring' (*The Times* 19 June 1876). The Lord Chief Justice took a similar line saying that up to now unlawful intercourse led to the birth of offspring and so the removal of this restraint 'may remove one of the restraints on vice and one of the safeguards on morality' (Francome 1984a: 36). The neo-Malthusians were initially found guilty but freed on appeal; the publicity caused sales of the book to increase from around 1,000 a year before the trial to 125,000 copies between March and June 1877. From that time onwards condoms were available: these were thicker than they are nowadays and were washed and reused.

Before the First World War the neo-Malthusians were the only group promoting contraception; the socialists were opposed. Marx called Malthus's work a 'shameless plagiarism' and the Socialists believed the way to eradicate poverty was by a wholesale change in the social order (Francome 1984a: 43). During the war it was agreed that after it the neo-Malthusians would set up a new organisation promoting contraception on its own merits and not as a cure for poverty. In 1921, Lord Dawson, the King's physician, called for the Church of England to accept birth control, and in 1930 he was successful. In 1921 Marie Stopes opened the country's first birth control clinic. In the 1920s the Catholic opposition to contraception became more active under an organisation called the League for National Life. Sutherland, its leader, said the propaganda for birth control had spread through the country 'until it reached the invisible and invincible frontiers of the Catholic church'. The arguments used at the time were similar to those still used against abortion today. They argued that birth control was dangerous and led to sterility, that it led to a breakdown in morality, that it was 'unashamed war upon babies' and would destroy the family. Another argument was that many 'great men' would not have been born. To counter this, the US activist Dr Robinson said society would have been prevented much misery if the mothers of Dillinger, Hitler, Al Capone, Goering and Oswald Mosley had used birth control (Francome 1984a: 89). In 1947 Sutherland examined the reasons why the movement against contraception failed: 'We witnessed the medical profession betray its trust, we saw the white flag hoisted over Lambeth Palace, we were in Whitehall in 1931 when the Ministry of Health first permitted advice of birth control to be given in antenatal clinics.

We complete this brief discussion of contraception with comments from Hayley Blackburn of the FPA (personal communication):

The Family Planning Association began life in 1930 as the National Birth Control Council, with 20 clinics, which provided advice 'so that married people may space or limit their families and thus mitigate the evils of ill-health and poverty'. It campaigned for contraception to be provided free of charge and by local authorities, and ran clinics itself in areas where they were not available. The organisation changed its name to the Family Planning Association in 1939 (and became FPA in 1998). In 1948 the National Health Service was created. However, family planning services were not included in the NHS so FPA continued to run its clinics until the 1970s.

Although attitudes towards contraception improved throughout the 1950s, it was not until FPA's silver jubilee that a health minister ever visited the organisation. In 1955, Mr Iain Macleod, Minister of Health, made a highly publicised visit to FPA, praising the 'admirable work' of the organisation. This was the first time the work of FPA had ever been mentioned on the BBC. However, prejudice against contraception continued and in 1960, FPA's first advert on the London Underground was withdrawn by the British Transport Commission after complaints from members of the public.

FPA played a significant role in the development of the combined oral contraceptive and it was approved by FPA's Medical Advisory Council for use in FPA clinics in 1961.

After family planning services were incorporated into the NHS in 1974, FPA handed all of its 1,000 clinics over to the NHS. Since then, the organisation has focused on campaigning and providing education, training and advice. FPA now runs a comprehensive information service, Sexual Health Direct, funded by the Department of Health, including a national telephone helpline, which responds to around 80,000 queries each year on a wide range of sexual health issues. The organisation also produces a variety of publications to support professionals and the public, and provides resources including training courses for those involved in delivering sexual health services. FPA has developed and delivers community-based education programmes for parents and for young people. FPA also runs two annual awareness campaigns: Contraceptive Awareness Week in February and Sexual Health Week in August.

Abortion was made illegal in 1803 in large part to protect the health of women. There were two other acts before the 1861 Offences Against the Person Act which are still in force today, although heavily amended. The Offences Against the Person Act stated that a person should not 'unlawfully' end a pregnancy. This implied there were lawful conditions, for example to save the woman's life; this was ambiguous. The first call for legal abortion was that of Stella Browne in 1915 who argued that as contraception was not perfect it needed a backup, that young people were not well educated, that ignorance should not be punished, and that it left people open to blackmail (Francome 1984a: 64). Shortly after her article was published there were reports of French women raped and impregnated by German soldiers. The *British Medical Journal* noted that there was sympathy for such women to be able to obtain abortions (20 March 1915). In 1929 the Infant Life Preservation Act was passed. This act addressed infanticide and made it illegal to kill a child in the process of being born. It made an exception to save the woman's life and several years later was regarded as having relevance to the Abortion Act. The Abortion Law Reform Association (ALRA) was founded in 1936 and had its first success in 1938 when a girl of 14 was raped and became pregnant. The doctor concerned, Aleck Bourne, was told 'she was with two girl friends, who ran off and left her, and she was held down by five men and twice assaulted'. He was then asked 'whether someone of your standing were prepared to risk a cause célèbre and undertake the operation in hospital'. Bourne agreed 'I have done this before and have not the slightest hesitation in doing it again' (Francome 1984a: 70). He was tried under the 1861 act and acquitted; from that time onwards abortion was considered legal for rape. The judge made the point that a doctor who, for religious reasons, did not perform an abortion to save a woman's life: 'would be in great peril of being brought before this court on a charge of manslaughter for negligence' (Francome 1984a: 70).

There were several bills to change the law: one decision that had to be made was whether to aim for reform of the law or have it repealed to give women the right to choose. A tea party at the House of Lords (12 February 1964) led to the ALRA chair writing: 'The Association would not stand a chance of getting a (repeal) bill introduced in the present climate of opinion.' So the aim became to reform the law. There is a tradition of a free vote in the House on such a bill and David Steel was third in the ballot. His bill was passed on 27 Oct 1967 and came into operation six months later. One debate towards the end of the discussions was on the degree of risk to the pregnant woman necessary for a legal abortion. The Lord Chief Justice, who was generally opposed to the bill proposed, 'Abortion should be legal if the risk to life or the risk of injury to health was greater by continuing the pregnancy rather than terminating it.' The Home Office said the wording was not a profound change. Norman St John Stevas, the prominent Catholic MP, said that if abortion was as safe as the reformers claimed then abortion would always be legal (Francome 1984a: 99). At the time of the 1967 act, the time limit for abortion was set by the Infant Life Preservation Act at 28 weeks. This act did not apply to Scotland where there was consequently no upper limit. In 1990 the time limit was reduced to 24 weeks with certain exceptions such as severe deformity. It came into effect on 1 April 1991 (Francome 2004a: 34).

In the early days of the act the number of abortions grew and the number of deaths from unsafe abortions rapidly fell. In 1980 the rate of abortions was 12.8 in England and Wales and 8.4 in Scotland (Francome 1984a: 129). The 2006 figures show there were 193,700 abortions on indigenous women which was a rate of 18.3 abortions per thousand women aged 15–45 in England and Wales. There were signs that abortions were being carried out earlier with 68% being carried out less than ten weeks' gestation – a 22% increase since 2002 (Ward 2007a). There were particular difficulties in obtaining abortions in the Midlands, which led to the formation of the Birmingham (later British) Pregnancy Advisory Service (BPAS). This organisation was formed in 1968 and by 2002 had a national network of 12 clinics and day care units supported by 35 consultation centres. The organisation carried out over 40,000 abortions a year and over two-thirds of these were carried out on an agency basis, paid for by the NHS but provided free to the women. BPAS was represented on the working party which developed the Royal College of Obstetricians and Gynaecologists' evidence-based guidelines *The Care of Women Requesting Induced Abortion*.

The other major charity carrying out abortions in the UK is Marie Stopes International (MSI) which operates in over 40 countries. In 2005 it served nearly 5 million clients and prevented an estimated 11,000 women's deaths.

The law in the UK does not give women the right to choose an abortion; this is of concern to a number of people who point out that a woman may seek referral from a general practitioner who is anti-abortion and therefore have problems of access. In 2007 the Medical Ethics Committee of the British Medical Association called for a change in the law so there would be no medical criteria during the first trimester, that the signature of only one doctor would be needed, that trained midwives could carry out both medical and surgical abortions, and that there would be no need for the premises to be approved. This change would bring the British law more into line with that of many other countries which now give women abortion on request. Following this announcement the government launched an inquiry into the impact of scientific developments on the abortion law. This led one commentator to say: 'The committee could end up recommending making early abortion easier to obtain and lowering the time limit' (Ward 2007b).

## Conclusion

We have seen that the distinctions between Eastern Europe and the rest of the countries of Europe are marked. There are signs that change is occurring and we may expect the number of abortions to decline as modern contraception becomes more widely available. There are wide variations in abortion rates even within Western Europe although some countries have shown signs of progress. The abortion rate in Italy, for example, declined by a third in the years 1980–1999, abortions are down by a quarter in Denmark, by a fifth in Finland and also reduced in France and Sweden.

# ASIA

*EVERY DAY PREGNANT WOMEN GO TO THE
CHURCH NOT ONLY TO PRAY BUT TO BUY
ABORTION DRUGS FROM THE DOZENS OF
STALLS THAT SURROUND IT.*

**CH Conde 2005**

U nsafe abortion is a major cause of maternal morbidity and mortality in Asia. Overall the World Health Organization (WHO 2004) estimates that in the year 2000 the continent had 10.5 million unsafe abortions and that there were 13 unsafe abortions per thousand women aged 15–44. These rates would have been much higher if it were not for the fact that abortion is legal on request in China. Unsafe abortions accounted for 34,000 deaths in 2000, which is 13% of pregnancy-related deaths (WHO 2004: 13). Asia's population growth has reduced in recent years. In the period 1970–1975 there were 5.1 children per woman. This fell to 2.9 per woman in the period 1990–1995 and to 2.7 in 1995–2000 (UN 2004: 29). At this rate it is nearing replacement rate. However, the overall figure is reduced by the significance of China. The UN region of Asia includes many countries in the Middle East and countries such as Turkey which many would consider to be in Europe. For consistency with other researchers we shall follow the UN geographical regions. This further divides Asia into four sub-regions: Eastern, South Central, South Eastern and Western. Countries in the region with over 300,000 people are as follows:

- **Eastern Asia**   China (and Hong Kong), Democratic People's Republic of Korea, Japan, Mongolia, Republic of Korea

- **South Central Asia**   Afghanistan, Bangladesh, Bhutan, India, Iran (Islamic Republic of), Kazakhstan, Kyrgyzstan, Nepal, Pakistan, Sri Lanka, Tajikistan, Turkmenistan, Uzbekistan

- **South Eastern Asia**   Brunei Darussalam, Cambodia, East Timor, Indonesia, Lao People's Democratic Republic, Malaysia, Myanmar, Philippines, Singapore, Thailand, Vietnam

- **Western Asia**   Armenia, Azerbaijan, Bahrain, Cyprus, Georgia, Iraq, Israel, Jordan, Kuwait, Lebanon, Occupied Palestinian Territory, Oman, Qatar, Saudi Arabia, Syrian Arab Republic, Turkey, United Arab Emirates, Yemen.

The overall population of Asia is 3.9 billion and is expected to increase to 5.2 billion by 2050. In 2003 the overall birth rate was 19 per thousand and the death rate eight per thousand, a rate of natural increase of 1.1%. In 2005 the total fertility rate was 2.4. Family size varies greatly between the countries with 2005 figures of 1.2 in South Korea and 7.8 in Afghanistan (Wright 2006: 481).

The number of unsafe abortions also varies greatly according to WHO figures. In Eastern Asia legalisation of abortion has meant that there are a negligible number of unsafe abortions. However, in South Central Asia there are yearly 7.2 million abortions, and 22 unsafe abortions per thousand women aged 15–44. In South Eastern Asia there are 21 unsafe abortions per thousand women aged 15–44. Western Asia has a much lower figure, at 12 per thousand women of childbearing age. In South East Asia almost one in five (19%) of maternal deaths are due to unsafe abortion. As measured by the number of unsafe abortion deaths per 100,000 live births, the highest rate is 70, in South Central Asia (WHO 2004: 13).

The regional offices of the International Planned Parenthood Federation (IPPF) in South Asia and in South Eastern Asia and Oceania have stated that their goal is to make abortion rare, safe, legal and available, and to move forward the liberalisation of abortion services. This is a challenge, especially in regard to expanding access to vulnerable and marginalised women, couples, unmarried women and young people. The IPPF regional offices identify the following problems in improving services:

- reduced efforts to address unsafe abortion due to legal, political, cultural and religious barriers in the region
- donor restrictions on funding related to abortion – notably the US gag rule
- poor data and documentation of abortion-related issues resulting in limited availability of evidence-based documents for advocating with governments.

Many countries in Asia encounter a lack of capacity in implementing clinical abortion-related services and in effectively advocating the right to access safe abortion. Young people and unmarried women are particularly under served. Where abortion laws are the least permissive, such as in the Philippines, Myanmar, Lao PDR and the Pacific Islands, IPPF suggests it is critical to open unsafe abortion to public debate and address the social and cultural mores that stigmatise women who have had abortions (personal communication).

Unsafe abortion continues to be one of the most easily preventable causes of maternal mortality. In 2003, reducing the maternal mortality rate (MMR) was identified as a cross-cutting regional challenge, with levels of MMR ranging from 120 in Iran to 1,500 in Nepal. Across Asia, abortion remains a controversial issue because of social, cultural and religious factors, which often translate into discrimination against women. The situation is exacerbated in South Asia, where entrenched gender discrimination and inequity deny women their bodily integrity, the right to control their fertility owing to poor access to reproductive health services, lack of awareness of the implications of unsafe abortion, and the inability to make informed decisions on abortion and related services.

A report for the UN by leading Arab researchers became the subject of impassioned debate in 2002. They found that development was being undermined by failings on three major issues: civil and political freedom, knowledge production and dissemination, and the empowerment of women. The failure of women to gain equality might be linked to continued high fertility: the average total fertility rate for the Arab world was 3.4 children per woman, which was high compared with the world average of 2.7 but is a great reduction from the averages of over six children found in the previous generation (DeJong et al. 2005; Fargues 2005: 43). One of the major reasons for the change has been the rising age of marriage. Three-quarters of women in the 1950 birth cohort married under the age of 20 compared with just one-third in the 1970 cohort. Mean age of marriage has risen from under 20 to over 25 in just one generation. Increasing length of education is a crucial factor. The proportion of married women in the labour force in Arab countries was one-third in 2000 and it is still not wholly acceptable for married Arab women to work outside the home. However, patriarchal practices are diminishing and changes are clearly going to continue. For larger nations, let us consider the situation country by country.

## Afghanistan

The population was estimated at 31.1 million in 2006. Over the period 2000–2005 life expectancy at birth was only 43 years. The population is 84% Sunni Muslim and 15% Shia with only 1% being of other religion. In the year 2003 the birth rate was 41 per thousand and the death rate 17 per thousand, a rate of natural increase of 2.4%. In 2005 the average woman had 7.8 children and if trends continue the population will more than double, to 69.5 million, by the year 2050.

The country has endured invasions from the Soviet Union and the UK/USA. These invasions prevented improvements in health for the local population. The health problems are such that one estimate suggests that, in Afghanistan, there is a maternal death in childbirth every 20 minutes. The infant mortality rate during 2000 to 2005 was 149, and estimates are that one in five children dies before the age of 5. This means that for every thousand mothers there would be around 1,600 early childhood deaths.

At one time the country had a law opposing abortion. It was allowed only to save the life of the woman. A person procuring an abortion even at the wish of the woman by 'beating or any other harmful means' was to be sentenced to a term of imprisonment of up to seven years. This was a relatively modest sentence compared with some other countries in the region.

A problem for the country's family health services came with the election of George Bush. He reinstated the gag rule in January 2001. As we have seen he prohibited US funds going to abortion-related non-governmental organisations. However, an important liberalisation of the position occurred in August 2005 when seven family planning centres opened, but the executive director of the Afghan Family Guidance Association (AFGA) stated that outside the capital there is little activity.

## Bangladesh

In 1901 the area of East Bengal had a population of 29 million. The name changed to East Pakistan and in 1951 the population of the area had risen to 44 million. It rose to 87 million by 1981; the population had tripled in only 80 years. By 2006 the population estimate was 147.4 million with a total fertility rate of 3.1 children per woman in 2005. Contraceptive use increased from 36% in married and cohabiting women in 1990 to 54% in the year 2000; of these, 43% were modern methods of contraception (UN 2004: 57). Bangladesh remains one of the few countries where female life expectancy at birth is lower than that of males, with levels of maternal mortality rates remaining unacceptably high. The Bangladesh Bureau of Statistics 2000 data have also shown that one-fifth (21%) of maternal deaths were due to complications from abortion. Other studies have confirmed that the major causes of maternal death in the country include postpartum haemorrhage, eclampsia and complications of unsafe abortions.

Overall, the estimated lifetime risk of dying from pregnancy and childbirth-related causes in Bangladesh is estimated to be 100 times higher than in the developed countries. A number of population-based studies have shown that abortion complications are responsible for nearly a quarter of deaths of women (Bangladesh Bureau of Statistics 2000).

In 1978 abortion deaths accounted for 26% of pregnancy-related deaths. This led in 1979 to a government circular including menstrual regulation in the national family planning programme; a national programme was developed to train doctors and paramedics to provide this in all public health facilities. Subsequently, menstrual regulation as a safe abortion service was included as part of the reproductive health package of services within the national Health and Population Sector Programme and the 1998–2003 five-year national health programme of the government. Following the completion of this five-year plan, the national Health, Nutrition and Population Sector Plan 2004–2007 addressed the menstrual regulation issues with the same priorities as before.

Government rules officially limit menstrual regulation service provision to the first two weeks following a missed menstrual period where pregnancy cannot yet be diagnosed reliably by either pelvic examination or urine test. In practice, menstrual regulation services are officially sanctioned and provided within two to four weeks of a missed period (i.e. 6–8 weeks since last menstrual period) and, if necessary, up to six weeks since the missed period.

IPPF documents suggest that despite the recorded success stories of a government-supported menstrual regulation programme across a largely conservative Muslim country, universal access to safe abortion (or menstrual regulation) services in Bangladesh remains a distant dream. This is because the take-up and utilisation of menstrual regulation services remains consistently low outside conurbations. A range of access problems, including lack of knowledge of the availability of services, low affordability (high fees and transport costs) and women's lack of decision-making power, limit their ability to control their fertility.

Entrenched gender inequality and discrimination limit women's awareness of their rights and knowledge about their entitlement to available services, and restrict their ability to access health care services. As a result, clandestine abortions conducted in unhygienic conditions by untrained practitioners continue to lead to high maternal mortality rates.

## China

The population was estimated to be 1,313.9 million in 1996. In the period 2000–2005 the total fertility rate was 1.7 and the average life expectancy was 72 years. This had increased from 59 in 1970. The infant mortality rate was 34 per thousand live births. In 2003 the birth rate was 13 per thousand, and the death rate seven per thousand, a rate of natural increase of 0.6%. On current trends the population is expected to increase slightly to 1,395.2 million by the year 2050 (Wright 2006: 482). The capital, Beijing, has a population of 11.2 million. The largest city is Shanghai, with a population of 13.6 million. China has no official religion but traditionally there was Taoism and Buddhism. Christians comprise 3–4% of the population and Muslims 1–2% (Wright 2006: 555).

Abortion was legalised by a directive from the minister of health in 1957. Peiping University president Ma Ying-Chu was quoted in the *New York Times* (28 July 1957) as saying that China must attempt to limit its population or face defeat in efforts to industrialise and raise living standards. In a special article Chen Muhua, a vice-president of the People's Republic, stated that China's population had risen from 540 million in 1949 to 975 million in 1978. He reported the success in reducing the crude birth rate from 40 per thousand population in the 1960s to 18.4 in 1978. The rate of natural increase had dropped from 23.4 to 12.1 per thousand between 1971 and 1978. He said that the aim was to get to zero population growth by the year 2000. He noted that amongst the 17.4 million births, 5.2 million were a third child or subsequent, and if these could be eliminated the rate of natural increase would be reduced to only seven per thousand. Muhua also drew attention to the incentives to persuade people to have just one child. These included a stipend until the child was 14 years old and priority in schools and jobs. He commented that the Marxist states had been overcritical of Malthus and argued that a rapidly expanding population was detrimental to capital accumulation and affected the standard of living.

China introduced its one child policy in 1979. The official position is that this was not to be facilitated by coercion and that forced abortion and sterilisation were against the law. However, the abortion rate rose. During the period 1973–1978 the number of abortions was relatively stable and increased only marginally from 5.1 million to 5.2 million. Numbers then rose over the next five years to a peak of 14.4 million in 1983 before decreasing and stabilising at around 10 million abortions a year. Although the official position is that women should not be coerced into abortion, the Western media has reported numerous cases where women have been forced to have terminations against their will. This may be due to over-zealous local authorities going beyond the national directives. An example was reported by Associated Press (2005). In Linyi, a city of over 10 million people situated around 400 miles south-east of Beijing, local authorities reportedly raided the homes of families with two children and sterilised one of the parents. The article also said that women who were pregnant with a third child were forced to have an abortion. Activists on the issue were making attempts at legal redress.

The one child policy seems to be much more observed in the urban areas. In rural districts the policy has been less emphatically followed. Even in the urban areas the policy is not now so fixed. Chinese students in London from single child families told us that if they married another only child they would then be 'allowed' to have two children.

One problem identified by the Chinese news agency Xinhua is that many people when obliged to have only one child have preferred it to be male, so that by 2006 it was estimated that 117 boys were born for every 100 girls. Two years earlier there was a report that of 31 provinces, regions and municipalities in China, all but seven had at least 110 baby boys born to 100 baby girls. This led to a 'care for girls' campaign supported by the authorities. Zhao Baigo commented that the aim was to have a normal sex ratio by 2010 (Xinhua 2004). One of the policies it addressed was the concern of some that they would not have a son to look after them in old age. The plan was that those reaching the age of 60 could receive state help.

## India

The population was estimated at 1,095 million in 2006. The natural increase rate is 1.7%, which, it is estimated, will lead to a population of 1,531 million by 2050. The average woman has 3.0 children. In the years 2000–2005 infant mortality was 68 per thousand births. The capital, New Delhi, had a population of 11.7 million in 2006. Mumbai (greater Bombay) was larger at 18 million. The population is 81% Hindu, 12% Muslim, 2% Christian and 2% Sikh (Wright 2006: 591).

India in some ways mirrors China in terms of government concern with overpopulation. In 1951 it sponsored a birth control programme and since that time has continued to promote various measures. One was sterilisation, which was particularly encouraged for almost two years until March 1977. During this period 10 million people received a vasectomy or tubal ligation. Many of these operations were compulsory for parents of three or more children. This programme led to the defeat of the government of Mrs Ghandi and was drastically cut back. The National Family Health Survey in 1989–1990 investigated contraceptive methods and found that 34% of women chose a permanent method of contraception, 12% other methods, and 52% of women continued not to employ any contraceptive method. This changed and in the year 2000 three in five (60%) married women were using contraception. There is also evidence that condoms are being promoted in the country in response to the HIV/AIDs prevention programme; 80% of India's £12 billion five-year programme is dedicated to promoting condoms. There is some opposition, however, and Hindu nationalists have been campaigning for the elimination of sex education in many schools and have suggested teaching teenagers yoga instead (Page 2007a).

The Indian Penal Code 1862 and the Code of Criminal Procedure 1898 had their origins in the British Offences Against the Person Act 1861 Act which made abortion illegal except to save the life of the woman. The high number of unsafe abortions leading to maternal mortality in 1964 led to a re-evaluation of the situation with the government-appointed Shah Committee:

> Doctors frequently came across gravely ill or dying women who had taken recourse to unsafe abortions. They realized that the majority of women seeking abortion were married and under no socio-cultural pressure to conceal their pregnancies and that decriminalizing abortion would encourage women to seek abortion services in legal and safe settings (Hirve 2004: 114).

The Shah committee carried out a comprehensive review of the law on both medical and compassionate grounds and in 1966 called for a legalising of abortion. It led to the Medical Termination of Pregnancy Act (1971) and legalised abortion throughout India except in the states of Jammu and Kashmir. The law allowed doctors to carry out an abortion on a variety of grounds including rape and incest and grave risk to the physical or mental health of the woman in her actual or foreseeable environment, such as when the pregnancy results from contraceptive failure, or on humanitarian grounds. It also allowed abortion for fetal abnormality. The operation can take place in any hospital maintained by the government but requires approval or certification of any facility in the private sector. For abortions up to 12 weeks' gestation only one doctor's signature is needed but for 12–20 weeks two are needed, except in an emergency (Hirve 2004: 115). Although abortion is legally available in a variety of situations the doctor still has the final authority.

In 1982 SM Dasgupta told a population control conference that nearly four million illegal abortions were carried out each year. He called for further liberalisation of the law and for women to have abortion on request (*Guardian* 17 February 1982). In the early years of the act, until 1986, there was only a slight increase in the number of approved abortion facilities and around a 10% increase in the number of abortions performed in them. Then in the late 1980s and the 1990s there was a reduction in the number of abortions carried out in approved facilities. In 1989, of the estimated 5.3 million abortions induced in India, 4.7 million (87%) took place outside approved health care facilities and were therefore potentially unsafe (Population Information Program 2007). Even in the mid-1990s less than 10% of the estimated total number of abortions was reported to the government. The fact that they were not registered does not mean they were necessarily unsafe. The Indian parliament tried to take more control of the situation with new measures including the Medical Termination of Pregnancy (Amendment) Act 2002. It improved some of the bureaucracy surrounding registration and, for example, facilities were no longer required to have on-site capability of managing emergency complications (Hirve 2004: 116).

In 2000, the National Population Policy of India was instituted to promote family planning; it also recognised the importance of providing safe abortion facilities. However, there are still obstacles for a woman seeking an abortion. A woman has to justify the fact that she, for example, had contraceptive failure. Also, although the act does not deny care to the single or the widowed, divorced and separated, it uses the phrase 'where any pregnancy occurs as a result of failure of any device or method used by any "married" woman or her husband for the purpose of limiting the number of children' (Hirve 2004: 117). Some activists have argued for changing 'married women' to 'all women'. This has not been taken up as 'it would imply tacit recognition and sanction of sexual relations among those who are unmarried or were previously married' (Hirve 2004: 117).

India is also similar to China in there being evidence of abortion used for sex selection. This was especially the case during the 1970s and 1980s. One of the advertisements read 'Invest 500 rupees (for a sex test) now and save 50,000 rupees (for a dowry) later'. Mrs Renuka Chowdhury, the Minister of State for Women and Child Development stated that the number of girls per thousand boys was 945 in 1991 but fell to 927 in 2001 (Page 2007b). In 2002 the government banned abortion for the purpose of sex selection. In 2006 the government launched a national campaign with the slogan 'My strength, my daughter'. *The Times* carried a full page report in February 2007 on the problems of female infanticide and abortion:

> Police in central India have found 390 body parts from fetuses and newborn babies – thought to be unwanted girls – buried in the backyard of a Christian missionary hospital. Separately the Government said that it was setting up a network of girls' homes – dubbed the cradle scheme – in an effort to stop poor Indians from killing their daughters ... Boys in India are traditionally regarded as future breadwinners whereas girls are considered a financial burden (Page 2007b).

Mrs Chowdhury commented: 'It is a matter of international and national shame for us that India, with a growth of 9%, still kills its daughters.' She continued to say that they were telling the people that if they did not want girls they could place them for adoption in government-financed homes (Page 2007b). A number of proposals have been made to end sex selection. One was to allow abortion only up to 12 weeks' gestation – before the sex could be determined. This was countered with the argument that it would lead to illegal abortions in the case of pregnancies over 12 weeks.

The IPPF states (personal communication):

> Although government abortion facilities are free there are problems of access experienced by women living in isolated rural communities. The scenario is further compounded as the majority of abortion facilities are urban based, with only 1,800 out of the 20,000 Primary Health Centers providing abortion or abortion-related services (unpublished data). This is because of lack of resources to support fully functioning and equipped infrastructures and sufficient numbers of trained personnel. Government regulations exclude trained paramedical personnel from providing legal abortion services. Potential providers also face a number of problems in securing centre registration as required by the Medical Termination of Pregnancy Act. This leads to the creation of large numbers of non-registered abortion care centers, making quality control difficult. Additionally, the need to be near blood banks is another major deterrent to securing Medical Termination of Pregnancy registration, especially in rural areas. Often, the maneuvers required to obtain registration are frustrating, complicated, and time-consuming. The latest amendment to the Medical Termination of Pregnancy Act has greatly simplified the procedure. Appropriate authorities are now required to process registration applications within 3 months.

Abortion-seeking behavior in India demonstrates a universal need that cuts across communities, socio-economic status, cultures and religious affiliations. In India the demand for abortion services, largely but not exclusively by married women, indicates high levels of unmet need for contraception counselling and utilization. Pre-abortion and post-abortion counselling has to be seen as an integral aspect of a comprehensive programme of information, education and communication activities within a sexual and reproductive health and rights framework.

The Indian economy is growing and this will produce extra resources to improve services. It is also the case that misoprostol is widely available and so the government may have more success in improving services in the future.

## Indonesia

Indonesia has progressed a great deal. Life expectancy at birth increased from 47 in 1970 to 67 in the years 2000–2005. This suggests a great improvement in social life overall. Its population was estimated to be 245 million in July 2005 (Wright 2006: 594). Indonesia consists of over 18,000 islands with the five biggest being Jakarta, Sumatra, Kalimantan, Sulawesi and Irian Java. The population is 88% Muslim, 8% Christian, 2% Hindu and 1% Buddhist.

The government has been concerned with overpopulation for some time. In the mid-1980s it began providing free birth control services at public health centres. From 1988 it began to withdraw from this position and richer people began to make a contribution towards the costs; services were still largely free for the poor. In 1989 the UN gave its population award to the President of Indonesia in recognition of the support the country had given in encouraging contraception. Strictly speaking, abortion is illegal except to save the woman's life or for certain medical conditions, but there is evidence that some clinics are adopting a more liberal approach. One in Jakarta reported 500 abortions a month while another in Bali reported 7–10 abortions a day (Pangkahila and Pangkahila 2006).

Although the population is nominally Muslim, it does not seem that the sexual practices of the young follow the conservative behaviour of the past. There is a great amount of premarital sexual behaviour and teenage pregnancy is not uncommon, although exact figures are unavailable (Pangkahila and Pangkahila 2006). The government, however, is aiming for zero population growth in the near future.

IPPF local commentators write (personal communication):

Data collected by the Indonesian Member Association shows that about 80% of women who had an abortion were in the lower socio-economic groups. The data also observes that demand for abortion during the last three years has increased drastically despite severe public objections and police surveillance. Furthermore the country's socio-cultural and religious barriers also work to hinder abortion practice.

Indonesia has faced an economic crisis in the last decade, and among the social and health implications due to the crisis, unwanted pregnancies among the low socio-economic group is prominent (i.e. under $1 a day). This is due to:

(i) lack of contraceptives in the public sector clinics (less subsidies from the government)
(ii) inability of women, especially the poor, to pay for contraceptives
(iii) escalating prices of services

(iv) high cost of living index, and having enough children (Member Association study on abortion).

It is estimated that around 80% of unwanted pregnancies end in abortion, performed under safe or unsafe conditions. Safe abortion services are provided both in urban and rural areas by skilled providers (medical doctors), while unsafe abortions are provided by unskilled providers, such as traditional birth attendants and unskilled health providers.

At a 1998 workshop on post-abortion and maternal health care Prof. Dr Biran Affandi (Obs/Gyn), a Reproductive Health expert in Indonesia, expressed concern about the number of abortions performed by unskilled attendants. He said that in the urban areas 57% of medical doctors were skilled compared to 16% of midwives and 19% of traditional birth attendants. In the rural areas things were different with only 26% of medical doctors being skilled, an identical number of midwives and nearly a third (31%) of traditional birth attendants. (WHO 2006) He indicated that abortions by unskilled providers often lead to complications such as bleeding, pain and even death. The reason for women not seeking safe abortion is because the price of such services is $US 100–300. This is beyond the reach of the poor. Pre and post-abortion counselling is an important part of abortion services as it helps to reduce repeat abortion and unwanted pregnancy. In an abortion provider environment, the counselling section is often missing due to time constraints and the illegality of the practice.

The prevalence of abortion was estimated at about 1.3 million in the period 1995–2000. (Global Health Council 2002), yet abortion is completely prohibited by law, except to save a woman's life. (Center for Reproductive Rights 2005). Nevertheless, an estimated 80% of unwanted pregnancies end in abortion, performed either under safe or unsafe conditions. Unsafe abortion contributes to 14% of maternal mortality (WHO 2006). Although there are signs that Indonesia can improve its reproductive health care there is still much to do in this regard.

# Iran

The population was estimated at 68.7 million in 2006. In 2003 it was growing at a rate of 1.1% per year and the total fertility rate was 2.1 during the period 2000–2005 (Wright 2006: 482). The population was 89% Shia and 10% Sunni Muslims. The other 1% includes Baha'i, Christians, Jews and Zoroastrians (Wright 2006: 596).

Iranian women were amongst the first to work for equal rights in the early part of the nineteenth century. The leaders were repressed and sometimes executed. Until 1931 women could not seek divorce but this changed following pressure from women's organisations and in 1936 women gained entrance to Tehran University. Women gained the vote and the right to stand for election. Educational emancipation was such that by 1978 one-third of university students were female. Abortion was restricted by article 622 of the Islamic Punishment Law which allowed abortion only to save the life of the woman. The law stated that 'anyone who intentionally … causes an abortion should pay the blood money plus he/she would face one to three years in prison' (Jahani 2004). The blood money in question varied according to gestation but for a fetus that had just been implanted it was 20 dinars and then increased through the pregnancy.

After the revolution of 1979 and the increased importance of Islamic law, two stages of pregnancy were considered. Up to 120 days' gestation the fetus was considered not to have a soul. Once it was considered ensouled the pregnancy had a very different status. In March 2005 the agency France Presse reported that the increase in unsafe abortion pushed Iran's conservative leaders to consider a change in the law (Cabatu and Bonk 2005). Consequently on 5 April 2005 the parliament approved a liberalisation of the law to include abortion in certain cases including the possibility of birth defects. During the debate one member of parliament drew attention to the fact that abortion was not condemned by the Quran. Although the law was passed by parliament in Iran there are 12 clerical men appointed to a Council of Guardians who can overturn a law if they judge that it does not comply with Islamic principles. This occurred and the Council maintained: 'It is against sharia to abort children who would inflict a financial burden on the parents after birth due to mental or physical handicap.' A new law was passed on 31 May 2005 and approved by the Council of Guardians on 15 June: legal medical organisations specified 51 different medical problems for the woman and fetus which could justify abortion and others could be considered (Larijani and Zahedi 2006).

Iran's birth rate is relatively low, in large part owing to the presence of family planning clinics. Post-coital contraception is available, which helps in the case of rape or unexpected sexual intercourse. The family planning clinics by all accounts are supportive of women who have had illegal abortions. 'Health care providers do not feel compelled to report illegal abortions to authorities' (Larijani and Zahedi 2006). The movement to the use of prostaglandins for abortions instead of curettage has helped reduce the maternal mortality rate.

One of the practices in Iran that seems strange to many people but affects unwanted pregnancy is the practice of temporary marriage or *sigheh*. This practice applies only to Shias and not Sunnis and seems to have developed when people would be away from home for long periods and it was judged they could not be expected to forgo their sexual needs. President Rafsanjani said in 1990: 'Don't be promiscuous like the Westerners but use the God given solution of temporary marriage.' This led to some complaints of inequality as men could not only have four wives but also unlimited temporary marriages. Ten years later the *New York Times* told the story of Maryam and Karim who had a secret relationship which they carried out in Karim's mother's house for five years (2000). These temporary marriages can be as short or as long as people wish them to be. Maryam and Karim renewed theirs every six months. It meant they could engage in sexual activity quite legally and in keeping with their religion. Maryam had been married before and divorced and this meant she could undergo a temporary marriage without the permission of a male relative. In this case, after five years Karim decided to end the relationship and married a virgin. Maryam said that she now planned to look for a permanent marriage. This practice of temporary marriage allows the institutionalisation of less committed sexual relationships. Children of such relationships may not have the support of a committed father but with fertility control using contraception and abortion women may have the necessary control over their fertility.

# Iraq

The population was estimated at 26.7 million in 2006. During the period 2000–2005 the total fertility rate was 3.2 children per woman and life expectancy at birth was 59 years. The population is 60–65% Shia Muslim and 32–37% Sunni Muslim with Christians comprising around 3% (Wright 2006: 597). The capital, Baghdad, had a population of 3.2 million in the 1987 census. An instructive statistic shows the extent of the suffering nowadays of the people in Iraq in the domain of health. In 1970 both Iran and Iraq had an average lifespan of 55 years. By the period 2000–2005 the average Iranian lived an extra 11 years as compared with Iraqis (Wright 2006: 488). The war has had a disastrous effect on the health services; in the 18 months following the 2003 invasion more than a third of the facilities providing family planning facilities had been destroyed. It was estimated that the risk of death was 2.5 times the level before the invasion (Round Up 2005a). The figures for maternal mortality show that in 1989 there were 117 deaths per 100,000 births but that this figure had almost tripled to a death rate of 310 in 2002. Many clinics have been damaged and looted and contraceptive services have deteriorated (Majaj 2005).

# Israel

The population was 6.3 million in 2006.During the period 2000–2005 the average woman had 2.8 children and life expectancy was 80 years. The infant mortality rate was five per thousand (Wright 2006: 488). In 2003 the birth rate was 19 per thousand and the death rate six per thousand, giving a natural annual increase of 1.3% (Wright 2006: 482). The religious background is 80% Jewish, 15% Muslim (mainly Sunni), 2% Christian and 3% other religions (Wright 2006: 600).

One of the surprising things about the situation in Israel is that the passing of its abortion law became so contentious. It might be thought that given the role of Jews in liberalising the law throughout the world the country would have moved swiftly to abortion on request, particularly because in 1952 the District Court of Haifa ruled that abortion openly performed on bona fide medical grounds was legal. From that time onwards doctors were not prosecuted and in practice abortion was freely available from medical practitioners. The law in Israel is based on the 1977 Penal Code, clauses 312–21. In the lead-up to the act the issue of abortion divided Israeli society. The feminist groups pressed for women to have the right to choose. They were supported by those on the left but opposed by the orthodox religious groups, the right wing and the Israeli Society of Gynecologists. The *Jewish Chronicle* (19 March 1976) reported that a meeting of 500 rabbis proclaimed a worldwide day of prayer to prevent the liberalising law from coming into being as it could 'spell suicide for the nation'. This kind of argument has a long history and a variant was later used by the British Chief Rabbi (*Jewish Chronicle* 29 January 1982) when he argued that without abortion there would be 4 million Jewish Israelis rather than 3 million (Francome 1984a: 147). He drew comparisons to the murder of Jews by the Nazis. The weakness of this argument is that many Israeli women who had abortions would nevertheless go on to have the number of children they wanted when they felt the time and possibly their relationship was right. The right-wing nationalists argued for the need to increase the Jewish birth rate. Geula Cohen of Herut said: 'The only bill needed is one to encourage the birth rate, not to decrease it' (*Jewish Chronicle* 28 Jan 1977). She was opposed by the civil rights leader Shulamit Aloni: 'A woman's body is her own. It is not there to serve the army, the State or the nation.' The opposition of the gynaecologists seems to be largely because they objected to women feeling they had the right to make them carry out an abortion. When in June 1976 they were at a meeting at the Tel Aviv Hilton Hotel their meeting was invaded by 15 women calling 'We want abortions legalised' (Francome 1984a: 147).

The law that was passed in February 1977 was a compromise and permission was needed from a three-member committee consisting of two specialist doctors, one of whom must be a gynaecologist, and a social worker. One of these three must be a woman. The grounds for abortion were:

1) The woman was under 18 or over 40 years.
2) The pregnancy was the result of incest or other illegal activity such as rape or even potential illegitimacy.
3) The fetus was likely to be born with physical or mental defect.
4) The pregnancy was likely to endanger the life of the woman or cause her physical or mental injury.
5) The family or social circumstances of the woman were such that for her to have another baby would be seriously injurious to her or her children.

Political change gave the religious parties more power and led in 1980 to the fifth ground for abortion to be removed. A woman member of the Knesset (the parliament), who voted for the removal after originally supporting it, was quoted in the *New York Times*: 'I didn't change my views. I only changed my vote because it was put as a confidence vote in this government' (26 December 1979). Two years later, a leading Jerusalem gynaecologist was quoted as saying the change had had little effect because 'any woman who really wants to terminate her pregnancy will find a way to get it done' (*Jewish Chronicle* 19 March 1982).

There have been attempts to liberalise the law again. In 2004 a member of the Knesset, Teshef Chen, wanted the social clause returned because in order to get an abortion women had to lie and 'women should not be forced to lie to preserve religious, chauvinistic, patronising, archaic values'. In 2006 Zaheva Cal-On, of the Meretz Party, proposed a bill to abolish the Committee for Pregnancy Termination, on the grounds that rich women could bypass the committee by having their abortions performed privately. This bill was rejected by a large margin.

The actual number of abortions in 2005 was approximately 20,000 and only a few hundred were refused by the committee. The abortion rate per thousand women aged 15–45 shows some interesting trends. In 1979 it was 23.2 but then rose to a peak of 25.7 in 1984 despite the removal of the social clause from the law. Then the rate began to fall. In 1986 it was 18.4, in 1995 it was 14.3, and in 2005 only 11.8. This is less than half the peak 21 years earlier and suggests that contraceptive use had greatly improved (Johnston 2007b).

## Japan

The population was estimated at 127 million in 2006. Life expectancy, at 82 years, is the highest in the world with only Hong Kong being at the same level. The fertility rate per woman was only 1.3 during 2000–2005 (Wright 2006: 488). Most Japanese observe both Shinto and Buddhist rites. The capital, Tokyo, has a population of 7.8 million (Wright 2006: 606). Japan has by far the highest usage of condoms in the world. In 2000 almost half (46%) of Japanese couples used this as their method and it comprised three-quarters of Japanese contraceptive use; this contrasts with 5% worldwide (UN 2004: 60).

Japan was one of the first countries to liberalise abortion. In 1948 it passed the Eugenic Protection Law which allowed abortion until viability for a broad range of conditions including mental illness, hereditary diseases, leprosy, the health of the woman and rape. One requirement was that the woman should be examined by two doctors but this was removed in 1952. In 1949, the first year after the act, the number of abortions was 246,000. This doubled in the following year and rose to a peak in 1955 of 1,150,000 operations. Over the next 30 years it halved, which local observers put down as being due to improvement in contraceptive use. The time limit was reduced in 1976 to 23 weeks' gestation and on 1 January 1991 to 21 weeks. This latter change followed a case in 1988 where a doctor attempted to abort a 16-year-old girl but produced a live baby for which he neglected to care.

Dr Kunio Kitamura noted that in 2004 the number of abortions declined by 18,000 over the previous year to a total of 301,000 (2005). He proposed a number of reasons for this including that young people were engaging in less sexual activity, that some people were opting to have children instead, that sex education had improved and also the availability of emergency birth control if problems did arise.

## Korea, North (Democratic People's Republic)

The population was estimated at 23.1 million in 2006 and is expected to increase slightly to 25.0 million by the year 2050 (Wright 2006: 482). In the period 2000–2005 the fertility rate per woman was 2.0; life expectancy was 77 years. The birth rate was 18 per thousand population and the death rate was seven, a rate of natural increase of 1.1%. The religious background was Buddhism and Confucianism but autonomous religious activities are now almost non-existent (Wright 2006: 612). The country's capital is Pyongyang which has a population of 2.0 million. The local IPPF comments (personal communication):

According to the Reproductive Health survey of 1998 conducted by the Population Institute, the abortion rate among married women was 17.7 per 1000 women (MIAR: marital induced abortion rate). A majority of induced abortions (80.9%) was attributed to unwanted pregnancies. Other causes included limiting the number of children, birth spacing and contraceptive failure. From 1998 to 2001, the MIAR declined from 17.7 to 11.1 following efforts to promote FP services (the current contraceptive prevalence rate is 67% and the most common contraceptive methods are IUD followed by oral contraceptives, spermicides and condoms). According to the 2002 RH survey, the gestational age (GA) at the time of abortion was 92.1% under 12 weeks, 6.3% at 132–0 weeks, and 1.6% above 20 weeks.

The only legal method of induced abortion is surgical abortion provided by a trained medical doctor. Surgical abortion is associated with a rate of abortion related complications of 16.4 per 100 women (1998 RH survey). Complications are more common among women who had induced abortion at a late gestational age or who had repeated abortions. In most cases, the complications are attributed to the surgical procedure. There is no recent data on abortion complications and no breakdown on the nature of the complications. As we can see in the above data, not all abortion services, even legal, are safe.

It is therefore necessary to reduce the number of late GA abortions and repeat abortions, by promoting SRH services and creating a favorable environment for the provision of safe abortion services. The introduction of medical abortion will contribute to creating such an environment. Medical abortion will offer to women the rights to choice, confidentiality, convenience and safety. Medical abortion will contribute to decreasing the number of surgical abortion related complications.

In DPRK, health personnel of governmental or non-governmental institutions have no clear understanding, skills and knowledge of medical abortion and abortifacient drugs. As a non-governmental organization specialized in SRH services, KFP & MCHA will play a pioneer role in the introduction of medical abortion services.

## Korea, South (Republic)

The population of the country was estimated at 48.8 million in July 2006 (Wright 2006: 613). Life expectancy in the period 2000–2005 was 63 years and the fertility rate per woman was 1.2 children (Wright 2006: 482). In 2003 the birth rate per thousand was 13 and the death rate six, a rate of natural increase of 0.7%. If current trends continue the country, like China, is expected to reduce its population to 46.6 million in the year 2050 (Wright 2006: 482). The capital is Seoul with a population of 10.7 million. The religious background is 49% Christian, 47% Buddhist and 3% Confucianist. There is also a pervasive folk religion (Wright 2006: 613). Contraceptive use increased from 79% in married and cohabiting women in 1990 to 84% in the year 2000 and of these two-thirds (67%) were using modern methods of contraception (UN 2004: 57).

The Republic passed a law to make abortion illegal in 1953. In 1962 it instituted a family planning programme and although the law had not changed the number of abortions increased. The UN suggests that this was because physicians were willing to carry them out and the authorities were unwilling to prosecute. One reason for this might be that the government was concerned with overpopulation. The law was changed with some opposition and the Maternal and Child Health Law (30 January 1973) broadened the law.

In 1985 the National Fertility and Family Health Survey was published which provided data of the reasons for abortion. This showed three in five (61%) wished to prevent subsequent births, around one in seven (15%) were practising birth spacing and 7% had abortions to protect the mother's health; the other 17% gave a variety of reasons (UN 2006). So it seems that the primary reason for abortion was to prevent any further births. This contrasts with other countries such as the USA where abortion is more usual amongst single women who will probably have children at a later stage.

The total fertility rate was 4.7 in 1970 but steadily declined until in the period 2000–2005 it was only 1.2. Only two countries, Ukraine and Slovakia, had lower rates than this. In part the provision of free birth control may have been responsible. The reduction in family size to well below replacement rate led the government to move away from promoting a one-child family to promoting a two-child one.

## Malaysia

The population estimate for Malaysia was 24.3 million in 2006. Life expectancy at birth was 73 years during the period 2000–2005. This was an increase from 62 years in 1970. The infant mortality rate was ten and the average number of children per woman was 2.8 during the period 2000–2005 (Wright 2006: 482). The capital city is Kuala Lumpur with a population of 1.1 million. It has a wide variety of religions practised including Islam, Buddhism, Taoism, Hinduism, Christianity, Sikhism and Shamanism (Wright 2006: 626). Contraceptive use increased from 50% of married and cohabiting women in 1990 to three in five (61%) in the year 2000 (UN 2004: 57).

The Abortion Act 1967 was restrictive and abortion became illegal except to save a woman's life. The Malaysian Fertility and Family Survey carried out a survey of women's attitudes to abortion in 1974 which showed that 71% agreed with abortion for rape and 52% for the woman's health (Takeshita et al. 1986). In 1984 the government announced a new population policy aimed at promoting population growth as part of an emphasis on family life. This does not seem to have been successful. In 1989 there were concerns about illegal abortion and one estimate was that the abortion ratio was one to every three live births. The law was changed and the Penal Code Amendment Act provided for legal abortions to be performed safely under certain conditions. One of these conditions is that the 'continuance of the pregnancy would involve risk to the life of the pregnant woman or injury to the mental or physical health of the pregnant woman, greater than if the pregnancy were terminated'. This wording is clearly reproduced from the British Abortion Act 1967 and, as early abortion is always statistically safer than childbirth, there is a strong case for assuming that abortion is always legal. However, this point does not seem to have been made in the debate in Malaysia.

Whereas there are a variety of religions in Malaysia, the Muslims make a sizeable group and although the Koran says nothing about abortion, on 9 January 2003 the Muslim National Fatwa Council declared that cloning human fetuses was acceptable as long as the fetus was destroyed within 120 days. Ismail Abraham was quoted as saying that 120 days 'would be in keeping with the view in some sections of Islam that until a fetus reached four months it has no soul and therefore can be aborted' (Life Site News 2005). This reasoning could allow a Muslim woman to have an abortion in the early months of pregnancy without transgressing the rules of her faith. In contrast, the Roman Catholic clergy in Malaysia take a restrictive view, even of birth control: in 2003 Bishop Anthony Lee of the Diocese of Miri was quoted as saying he 'made it a number one priority to reiterate the Church's teaching against contraception and the whole culture of death' (Meaney 2003).

To investigate the ease of access to abortion in Malaysia a journalist telephoned six clinics at random. Three of these openly admitted that they would perform abortion but the other three were more reticent. One nurse said that one doctor carried out two abortions every day, further commenting: 'Some patients walk in wearing school uniform, accompanied by their boyfriend' (Palmdoc 2006). R Jegasothy of the Malaysian Medical Association made the point that over the previous ten years they had not had a single complaint that it could take up about an illegal abortion occurring, though it had received a few anonymous missives on the subject which could not lead to action. He suggested that doctors were filling a demand and that if they stopped, unskilled operators were likely to take over. He commented 'We do not now hear of women dying after inserting lalong or pineapple stalks' (Palmdoc 2006). Overall, abortion seems to be accepted as part of Malaysia's overall family planning policy.

## Myanmar (known as Burma until 1989)

The population was 47.3 million in 2006. In 2003 the birth rate was 19 and the death rate was 12, a rate of natural increase of 0.7% per year. During the period 2000–2005 the average woman had 2.3 children and life expectancy was 60 years (Wright 2006: 488). The religious background is 89% Buddhist, 4% Muslim, 4% Christian and 1% animist. The capital city is Yangon (formerly Rangoon) which had a population of 2.5 million according to the 1983 census. The second largest city is Mandalay with a population of over half a million (Wright 2006: 636). A local resident told us that the government wishes the population to reach 100 million. At the current rate this will take many years as on current trends the population will only reach 64.5 million by 2050 (Wright 2006: 483). Contraceptive use increased from one in ten married and cohabiting women in 1990 to four in ten in the year 2000 (UN 2004: 57).

Marie Stopes International Myanmar (MSIM) has been working in the country with a limited range of services since 1997. It provides help with HIV/AIDS and gives contraceptive assistance. Until 2006 this concentrated on 'birth spacing' but more recently people have been talking in terms of 'reproductive health'. Condoms are freely available in the country and are cheap at USD 0.15 each. Some agencies provide them free, presumably mainly to prevent the spread of HIV/AIDS. There was prejudice against the condom but our local informant tells us that the 'stigma has been reduced significantly in the past decade'. MSIM does not provide vasectomy nor tubal ligation as methods of contraception. The contraceptive pill is used, but recently there has been a shortage.

Abortion is illegal and local women go to China if they want a termination. In addition there is the Mao Tao Clinic, set up at the border town of Mae Sot, to which numerous women travel great distances for family planning and health care. One article said that in Burma there are 58 deaths each week from illegal abortion and gave the maternal mortality rates of Burma as 517 per 100,000 births compared with 200 in Thailand and 10 in Singapore (Aderson 2001). Although mifepristone (RU 486) is not yet legal, misoprostol is now available and if it became more widely known it could help reduce the death rates from illegal operations.

A local respondent told us that the media is controlled in the area of sexuality and, for example, 'illegitimate' (premarital or out of wedlock) pregnancies are not allowed to be portrayed in the local movies or the print media.

## Nepal

The population was estimated at 28.2 million in 2006 and it had a rate of natural increase of 2.2% per year in 2003. During the period 2000–2005 the total fertility rate was 3.5 children per woman. In 1970 the average length of life was 42 years and this increased to 61 years in the period 2000–2005. If current trends continue the population will rise to 50.8 million by 2050 (Wright 2006: 483). The population is 86% Hindu, 8% Buddhist and 4% Muslim (Wright 2006: 639). Contraceptive use increased from one in five (21%) married and cohabiting women in 1990 to one-third (33%) in the year 2000 and of these three in ten (29%) were modern methods of contraception (UN 2004: 57).

Women in Nepal have historically had a difficult time. In 2001 it was reported that Nepal was one of three countries in the world where the life expectancy of women was below that of men. The ratio of doctors to population was approximately five per 100,000 and of nurses about 22 per 100,000 (IPPF, personal communication). An article published in 2001 reported a Nepalese saying as 'To be born a daughter is ill fate' and it reported that four out of five women could not read and four out of five homes had no running water (Opesto 2001). An important study carried out in 1984, in five hospitals in and around Katmandu for a period of one year, found that the abortion providers were untrained and that 'as high as 50% of all maternal deaths in the study were due to abortion-related complications' (Thapa 2004). The 2001 Nepal Demographic and Health Survey found that one in five births were unwanted and a further 14% were mistimed. Illegal abortion was common and dangerous. One estimate was that around 4,000 Nepalese women died of abortion-related causes each year and that this constituted half of all maternal deaths (Uprety 1998). Fifty-four per cent of all hospital admissions were women with post-abortion complications.

The headline of an article released by BBC News was 'Abortion Nightmare in Nepal' (Singh 2004). This told how in the year 2000 Shanti Shresta had a problem with her pregnancy. She already had three children and was in her fourth month when she developed a migraine and took paracetamol. She said, 'I knew instinctively I was miscarrying ... my underclothes were drenched in blood.' She was taken to hospital by her landlady who had the responsibility of reporting such a miscarriage to the police. The police saw her as potentially aborting herself and at the hospital she had four armed policeman as guards. This was a waste of resources. 'I was so sick there was no reason for them to guard me. I could not run anywhere.' Her two teenage daughters were left with her husband who was a taxi driver. She was taken to prison and her 5-year-old son accompanied her. Although she was not unintelligent, she was illiterate. Consequently she could not read the paper the police presented to her, signed a confession and was sent to prison for 20 years. Her son was placed in care. Not surprisingly she was deeply traumatised by the event. Fortunately, when the law was changed in 2002 she was released. She said, 'I thought I was going to rot in jail. I never thought I would be released.' She had still not been reconciled with her son at the time of the report (Singh 2004).

This experience is by no means unique. In the 1990s nearly 100 women were in prison for carrying out abortions and in 1999 a nationwide study found that 20% of women in Nepalese jails had been convicted on charges of abortion or infanticide (Lak 2002; Shakya et al. 2004). Not one man was convicted for abortion-related activities in the whole history of the act (Uprety 1998). Given that a high percentage of pregnancies end in spontaneous abortion which cannot be proved, there were probably many women who were wrongly imprisoned even under a law which was later rescinded. On 14 March 2002 the national parliament of Nepal passed a law to legalise abortion for women under 12 weeks' gestation. For the period up to 18 weeks' gestation abortion was to be legal in the case of rape and incest. In the case of risk to the health of the woman or of a disabled fetus there was to be no time limit (Singh 2004). The law was not retrospective and, although some women were released early in April 2003, a report stated that over 50 women were still languishing in prison. In 2004 the king granted an amnesty for abortion offences (Singh 2004).

As to the future, in 2007 the IPPF reported (personal communication):

> There remain significant challenges to making safe abortion services widely available to women who need them. Nepal's topography, insufficient national level resource allocation to support medical services and entrenched gender inequality and discrimination, which prevent awareness of rights and ability to take up services, all work together to deny women access to safe abortion services.

> Demand for abortion needs to be understood in the context of unwanted pregnancies, contraceptive use and non-use and unmet needs. A micro level study conducted among married women in Kathmandu Valley found that nearly one third of rural women and more than one fifth of the urban women had experienced unwanted pregnancy at least once. More than one fifth of rural women and more than a quarter of urban women with unwanted pregnancies sought abortions. More than one third of both rural and urban

women said they would abort any unwanted pregnancies in the future. These facts indicate a potential for high demand for safe abortion services in Nepal. Doctors and gynecologists working in the Chitwan, Sunsari and Katmandu valleys estimate that two-thirds of women seek abortion services at least once during their childbearing years.

At present abortion services are largely concentrated in the urban centres. Additionally, there is an acute shortage of trained service providers who are able to provide the widest possible range of high quality abortion care services including post-abortion care. However, progress is being made and on 18 March 2004 the first comprehensive legal abortion services were opened at the Maternity Hospital in Kathmandu (Thapa 2004: 90). There was little knowledge about medical abortion but the easy availability of the drugs means that it is likely to have growing importance.

## Pakistan

The population estimate for Pakistan in 2006 was 165.8 million. Life expectancy in 2000–2005 was 63 years, increased from only 48 years in 1970. In 2000–2005 the total fertility rate was 4.0 children per woman. In 2003 the birth rate was 30 per thousand and the death rate nine per thousand. If current trends continue, the population is estimated to more than double to 348.7 million by the year 2050. The infant mortality rate was 79 per thousand live births between 2000 and 2005. This suggests that nearly one in three women will lose a child aged less than 1 year (Wright 2006: 488). The religious background is 77% Sunni Muslim, 20% Shia Muslim and 3% Christian, Hindu and other (Wright 2006: 646).

The Family Planning Association was set up in 1953. Since 1955 the government has instituted a series of five-year plans which have included reduction of population growth. Following the International Conference on Population and Development in Cairo in 1994, the government introduced programmes for birth control. The Population Welfare Division planned that over the five years 1993–1998 the population increase should reduce from 2.9% to 2.6% per annum. This would be accomplished in large part by improving the availability of family planning which would rise from 5% to 70% in the rural areas and 54% to 100% in the urban areas. This programme had moderate success but by the year 2003 the rate of increase had been reduced to 2.1% (Wright 2006: 483). Contraceptive use increased from one in eight (12%) married and cohabiting women in 1990 to one in three (33%) in the year 2000; 23% used modern methods of contraception (UN 2004: 57).

Other observers suggest progress has been limited in comparison with other countries, and one commented in 2005: 'Pakistan has one of the worst reproductive health records in Asia with reproductive health related diseases accounting for an estimated 12% of the total disease burden' (personal communication). A study of 171 (113 male and 58 female) general practitioners in the Sind region found only 25% reported providing reproductive health services in their practice. The study called for a doubling of public sector resource application over the five years to 2010 (Round Up 2005b). Marie Stopes International (MSI) began working in the country in 1992; Dr Laila Shah, its Medical Development Team Leader, told us (personal communication April 2007) 'Contraceptive prevalence rate is 36% in Pakistan due to poor access to family planning services, to the cost of these services, the fear of side-effects, myths and misconceptions about family planning methods, and religious beliefs.' However Dr Shah did note some causes for optimism in that:

Knowledge of family planning in Pakistan is high: In 2000–2001, an estimated 96% of currently married women were aware of at least one contraceptive method. Knowledge of how to obtain family planning methods is also high; for example, in 2000–2001, 76% of married women reported knowing a place where they could obtain a tubal ligation. Furthermore, condoms are freely available at affordable prices. The provision of family planning services in rural communities now rests with the Ministry of Health; community workers provide clients with oral contraceptives and condoms, while other family planning methods are available through networks of health centers. In urban areas, all modern methods are available through the public sector. However, the quality of care provided it is not yet optimal; the integration of family planning services within basic and essential health services is far from complete, and maintaining a consistent supply of contraceptives has been a continuing problem Nongovernmental organizations have helped to fill these gaps in family planning service and have played a vital role in improving family planning services' access among marginalized groups.

The Ministry of Population Welfare has attempted to address the challenge of meeting family planning needs by encouraging the private sector to deliver family planning services. The private sector provides more than 70% of all health care in Pakistan but has limited involvement in family planning, providing a smaller share of contraceptive coverage (20%) than either the public sector (54%) or nongovernmental organizations (26%) The private sector has generally adopted a social marketing approach, in which commercial techniques are adapted to the provision of family planning services, in an attempt to make products and services available and affordable to low-income groups.

The abortion law until 1990 was based on that developed by the British colonialists for India in 1860. This criminalised all abortions and if the woman was not 'quick with child' (under about four months) the woman or the practitioner could be sentenced for up to three years and/or a fine. It was increased to seven years for later abortions. The law continued to be in operation after independence. In 1989 the Pakistan Supreme Court found the law to be invalid as not in keeping with the principles of Islam. This led in 1990 to a new law which allows abortion for 'necessary treatment' but this is not clearly defined. It maintained the principle that there should be differences between abortion carried out before and after four months (quickening) in line with Islamist teaching that after this time the limbs and organs are formed and the fetus has a soul.

An investigation of the situation in Pakistan in 2002–2004 assessed that the abortion rate was 29 per thousand women and that overall there were 890,000 abortions a year. It discovered that pregnant women were often forced to visit illegal clinics run by midwives and that 23% of these abortions resulted in the women being hospitalised for complications. The report also suggested that men should become more involved in fertility control (Population Committee 2007). Dr Shah's comments were similar: she said that many doctors were unnecessarily frightened of the legal implications of carrying out abortions.

In the geographical areas where international groups are operating there is clearly much better access to a wide range of family planning services. Dr Shah told us: 'We are already providing FP services through 47 delivery services. These include all family planning methods including surgical ones, we also offer TSIC, which stands for Treatment for Septic and Incomplete Abortions, in all our centers.' So currently it seems that service is patchy and that more resources could greatly improve matters. However, the International Pregnancy Advice Service is providing training in manual vacuum aspiration to government and private doctors and as this early treatment accords with the tenets of the Muslim religion, it could prove acceptable. In addition, medical abortion is freely available using misoprostol, which is an anti-ulcer medicine. The government wants universal access to modern family planning methods by 2010 with a comprehensive network of services and a reduction of the population growth rate to 1.3% by the year 2020.

## Philippines

The population was 89.4 million in the middle of 2006 and increased at a rate of 2% during 2003. During the period 2000–2005 the average woman had 3.0 children. This is a reduction from 4.3 in 1985–1990 and 3.6 in 1995–2000 (Juaraz et al. 2005). Life expectancy at birth has been increasing and while in 1970 it was 57 years, in the period 2000–2005 it was 70 years (Wright 2006: 482, 488). The religious background is 83% Roman Catholic, 9% Protestant, 5% Muslim and 3% Buddhist and other (Wright 2006: 651). The abortion law in operation is the Revised Penal Code of 1930 which officially makes abortion illegal except to save the life of the woman.

The large Catholic majority has restricted the development of modern contraception. Dr Diego Danila of the Department of Health said that attempts to address unsafe abortions through initiatives such as more vigorous family planning are opposed by the Church. Conde, writing in the *International Herald Tribune*, said that Filipino politicians only speak about abortion to condemn it but that meanwhile 'more and more women are dying'. Fetuses are often dumped around the areas of churches. It is not clear to observers whether this is in order to secure eternal life for the supposed soul or whether it is to punish the Church for its hard-line attitude (Conde 2005).

Official estimates are that there are 400,000–500,000 unsafe abortions a year. The WHO puts the figure much higher at 800,000 abortions, the highest rate in Asia. Jean Marc Olive, the WHO local representative, estimates that 70% of unwanted pregnancies end in abortion. Over one-third (36%) of women are pregnant before marriage and the local 'pro life' group estimates that one in four pregnancies ends in abortion. Olive commented on a survey of attitudes to births: 'Families it seems would like at least one child less than they have' (Conde 2005).

An important study of the incidence of abortion was carried out by Juaraz and colleagues (2005). They obtained data from 1,658 hospitals and estimated that 78,900 people were hospitalised in a year for post-abortion care. They estimated 473,400 women had abortions, a rate of 27 per thousand women aged 15–44. One-third of the abortions were carried out by doctors or nurses and two-thirds by traditional practitioners. One-quarter of the hospitals in their study stated that the after-effects of abortion were one of the ten major causes of admission (Juaraz et al. 2005).

One of the centres for the distribution of abortifacient pills is the Quiapo Catholic Church in the capital, Manila. Conde says: 'Every day pregnant women go to the church not only to pray but to buy abortion drugs from the dozens of stalls that surround it.' The Church, he says, has 'become almost synonymous with abortion' (2005).

The anti-abortion leaders confirm the problem exists and are concerned about the high level of abortion. The leader of the Philippines 'pro life' group, a nun called Pilor Versoza, commented about the trade: 'We would assign volunteers to chase after women who had just bought from vendors and tell them about their options.' The group also put up a sign telling women there were alternatives to abortion; it was pulled down (Conde 2005). The best-selling abortifacient is Cytotec a drug (misoprostol) that was originally used to relieve ulcers. The drug was made illegal but is still on sale for a price of just below one dollar a pill. The right to life group says that they are smuggled in from South Korea and Bangkok.

Juaraz and colleagues comment that the high number of abortions in the country is part of a generally restrictive social and political climate. This has suppressed the development of modern forms of contraception and resulted in people using withdrawal and periodic abstinence. This leads to unwanted pregnancies and abortions. They suggest that there is a shortfall in services and that around half of women of reproductive age need effective contraception (2005).

## Saudi Arabia

The population was 27.0 million in 2006. In 2003 the birth rate was 37 per thousand and the death rate was six per thousand, a rate of natural increase of 3.1%. During the period 2000–2005 the total fertility rate was 3.8, and life expectancy was 72 years, which is 20 years higher than in 1970 (Wright 2006: 483). The religious background is almost 100% Muslim; most of these are Sunni and a fundamentalist version of Islam called Wahhabism. The capital city is Riyadh with a population of 1.8 million. Muslims from around the world are enjoined to visit the city of Mecca (630,000 population) at least once in their lifetime, if they can afford it. Medina (400,000 population) also has great religious importance (Wright 2006: 665).

The economy is to a large extent based on oil which constitutes 55% of its GDP and produces 80% of government income. There are no elections and the State closely adheres to the religion. Shops and restaurants close five times a day for prayers. No citizens are allowed to convert from Islam to another religion and other religions are not allowed to have public meetings. The society is strongly divided by gender and women in particular are subject to many restrictions. After their first menstrual cycle they must dress in a long black cloak called an abaya. They are neither officially allowed to drive cars nor ride bicycles, and this is enforced especially in the cities. Women are rarely allowed to testify in court and in the Sharia court the testimony of one man counts as equal to that of two women (USA Bureau of Democracy 2001). Women are not allowed to marry non-Muslims, but men may marry Christians and Jews. An unusual practice for Sunni Muslims is the practice of al-mesyar (or short daytime visit) marriages where the woman forgoes maintenance rights. There are no restrictions on the number of these that a man can contract and they are in addition to his official wives (Ottoway 2004). Women make up only 5% of the workforce but there was a slight liberalisation in 1997 when they were given authorisation to work in the hotel industry. Women are not allowed to travel alone nor with a man who is not a relative. They are not allowed to attend hospital unless accompanied by a male relative or with written permission and so clearly women cannot seek birth control or abortion. In the year 2000, 20 Saudi women obtained abortions abroad but this number declined to eight in the year 2005 (Johnston 2007c). There are external pressures for Saudi Arabia to liberalise its restrictions. These seem to be resisted and Amnesty International's report on the country reported a lack of co-operation from the authorities (2003).

## Sri Lanka

The population was 20.2 million in 2006. The population increase during 2003 was 1.0% and this relatively low level reflects the fact that the average woman has only 2.0 children. The population is 70% Buddhist, 15% Hindu, 8% Christian and 7% Muslim (Wright: 677). Sri Lanka was one of the first developing nations to understand the importance of investing in human resources and promoting gender equality. As a result, it has achieved health and education outcomes more consistent with those of high-income countries. It also liberalised its economy in the late 1970s ahead of other developing nations and maintained healthy economic growth despite a devastating 20-year civil conflict. Ninety per cent of Sri Lanka's poor continue to live in rural areas where access to basic services is limited.

Sri Lanka has undergone significant family change. The average age of marriage has increased. For women the average was 18.1 years in 1901 but increased to 24.6 years in 2000, a rise of 6.5 years. In 1998 education was made compulsory for the 5–14 years age group (da Silva 2003). An important development in the country occurred on 23 December 1997 when a population and reproductive health policy was approved by the National Health Council, chaired by the prime minister. It had eight goals which it hoped to achieve in 2008: to produce a stable population, safe maternity, sex equality, and responsible behaviour; increased responsibility towards the welfare of the elderly; promotion of the economic benefits of migrants; increased public awareness of health; and an improved population policy.

Marie Stopes International has been active in the country since 1973 and is in partnership with the local organisation Population Services Lanka. It aims to provide birth control services even in 'far flung villages' and reported that in 2002 66% of couples were using contraception and 44% were using modern methods (MSI 2007a).

As far as abortion is concerned the Penal Code of Sri Lanka is based on an 1883 law which permits abortion only to save a woman's life, making abortions performed under any other circumstances a criminal offence (da Silva 2003). Studies suggest that a high prevalence of abortion exists in the country. A US Aid report estimated that there were 150,000–170,000 a year and also commented that, although terminations are illegal, 'Abortion services have always been provided at private hospitals and clinics and occasionally at Government hospitals' (da Silva 2003). According to the Ministry of Health, women argue adverse emotional and psychological risks (e.g. severe mental depression, suicidal tendencies) to the wellbeing of the pregnant woman, and many are able to secure abortions at private or government hospitals. In these instances there is little or no government enforcement of the law. The Family Planning Association of Sri Lanka found that the majority of women seeking abortions are married and aged 25–39 (FPASL 2000). On 3 May 2006 anti-abortionists carried out a prayer vigil outside the Marie Stopes Centre in Colombo. They were led by Eshan Dias, President of Cultura Vitae who offered to pray for the doctors' conversion to Catholicism. Westen suggested that the Sri Lankans had been told that the UN wanted to depopulate the nation; it is not certain where such a fanciful notion came from (Westen 2006b).

IPPF commented in early 2007 (personal communication):

> The scenario for women from lower economic background is very different, as they are often forced to resort to illegal, unregulated services resulting in high mortality and morbidity. The illegal nature of the activity means that quality control mechanisms do not

exist to ensure that operations are carried out in safe and hygienic conditions, and that they are conducted by suitably qualified medical personnel. FPASL estimates that 10% of beds in gynecological units are occupied by women suffering from the after effects of unsafe abortions, and that post-abortion complications contribute to increasing maternal morbidity and mortality in Sri Lanka.

There have been attempts from parliamentarians, women's groups and others for reform of the law. IPPF report that the Medical Legal Society of Sri Lanka, the Ministry of Women's Affairs, the Ministry of Justice, and a number of women's groups are vigorously continuing their efforts to change the law (personal communication).

## Thailand

The population was estimated at 64.6 million in 2006. In the 1960s the average woman had over six children and the government started to sponsor family planning. Now the average woman has 1.9 children, below replacement level. Life expectancy at birth in the period 2000–2005 was 70 years, an increase from 58 years in 1970 (Wright 2006: 482). The population is 95% Buddhist and 4% Muslim (Wright: 687). The capital is Bangkok with a population of 5.9 million (1990 census). Contraceptive use was high at seven out of ten (71%) married and cohabiting women in 1990 and rose only slightly to 72% in 2000.

The abortion law in operation is based on sections 301–5 of the Thai Penal Code of 1956. Under it abortion is legal to protect the woman's health or as a result of rape or incest. The law is not, however, rigorously enforced and in the 1970s there were an estimated 300,000 illegal abortions (Population Division 2007a). The methods of abortion, it seems, have been either a traditional abortion massage or intra-uterine injections. Often complications would arise and in Ramathib hospital in Bangkok in 1981 one-quarter of all maternal deaths were due to illegal abortions performed outside a hospital (Population Division 2007a). Two feminists said that in 1993 there were an estimated 80,000 illegal abortions, which is a reduction of the estimate for the 1970s. They point out that smaller families tend to have more wealth and better education than larger families. Furthermore, liberalisation of attitudes toward fertility has led women to expect freedom in other areas of life (Lerdmaleewong and Francis 1998). In her book published in 2004, Whittaker estimated a higher number of unsafe abortions at 200,000–300,000 a year. Another in-depth study by Whittaker studied 164 women of reproductive age in rural areas and 19 others who had had an illegal abortion. She found wide support for a liberalisation of the law and that it was the poorer workers who were most at risk of complications because they were more likely to use untrained practitioners (Whittaker 2002). A 42-year-old woman told of her experience:

I first tried to induce abortion with an injection but after five days I had no menstruation so I paid to go to a midwife. She used an iron rod to abort. I was afraid so I returned home and instead asked my husband to massage and stamp on my stomach. I also bought some medicines that are very hot but still I did not abort (Aderson 2001).

With women facing such obstacles to safe treatment there is obviously pressure to change the law, but Whittaker proposes that while at one time the focus was on abortion and health, more recently the argument of reproductive rights is increasingly being used. The first moves toward liberalisation occurred in 1973 and in 1981 a bill was passed, but religious opposition prevented it from passing in the Senate. In recent years a network of groups have been working together to produce change. These include women's groups, journalists, academics and public health officials (Whittaker 2003, 2004).

It is not easy to assess accurately the levels and trends of abortion since the reported cases fluctuate with changes in coverage of reporting in the national statistics. The ratio peaked in 1992 at 44% live births and declined through the mid-1990s to 18% in 1998. This coincided with an increase in contraceptive use. The ratio started increasing again in 1999, probably due to the inclusion of private sector data in the national figures. In 2002 the ratio was 22, though it is suspected the 'corrected' data were far from accurate.

On recent evidence, Thailand needs extra resources put into increasing the awareness and practice of modern contraceptive techniques.

## Turkey

The population was 70.4 million in 2006. In 2003 the birth rate was 18 per thousand and the death rate was six per thousand, a rate of natural increase of 1.2%. On current trends it is expected that the population will increase to 97.8 million by the year 2050. Family size in Turkey has shown a rapid decline. In 1990–1995 there were 3.8 children per woman, but in the years 1995–2000 this had reduced to 2.5 and during the period 2000–2005 there was a further slight fall in births when the average woman had 2.4 children (Population Reference Bureau 2007). Life expectancy at birth was 69 years in 2000–2005, an increase from 57 years in 1970 (Wright 2006: 489). The median age of marriage is 19 years and 25% of women have their first baby by the age of 20 (Henshaw et al. 1999; Population Reference Bureau 2007). The country is 99.8% Muslim and the majority is Sunni Muslim; there are a small number of Jews and Christians. The capital is Ankara with a population of 2.7 million. The population of Istanbul is 7.3 million (Wright 2006: 690).

The country legalised contraception in the 1960s. There was a tendency for a high proportion of women to use traditional contraception; in 1968 24% of women were using withdrawal. In 1982 the government adopted a population policy to provide family planning as part of a plan to improve family health and welfare. From 1936 the abortion law restricted legal access to abortion to protecting the life or health of the woman or on the ground of fetal abnormality. The growing number of illegal abortions in early 1983 was a factor in leading to abortion and sterilisation being legalised on 24 May 1983 under the Population Planning Law. Abortion is now allowed on request in the first ten weeks of pregnancy under a law which also authorises general practitioners to terminate pregnancies. After ten weeks abortion is allowed to protect the life or health of the woman and for fetal impairment. After ten weeks two doctors must be involved in the decision: one must be an obstetrics and gynaecology specialist and the other a practitioner in another field. The woman must have her husband's consent for an abortion and single women must have the approval of their guardian (2007b).

In 1974 the Turkish Fertility Service found that 34% of Turkish women had had an abortion and in 1983 the Turkish Population and Health Survey found that 37% of those ever married had had at least one abortion. In 1993 there were 351,300 abortions but this figure must be an underestimate because it does not include single women. Even with under-recording the abortion rate was relatively high at 45 per thousand woman aged 15–49 in 1988 but it fell to 25 in 1993 and remained at this level in 1998 (Henshaw et al. 1999; Population Division 2007b). This reduction reflects well on improved contraceptive information during the period. In 2003 the Turkish Demographic and Health Survey pointed out that 24% of ever married women had had an abortion and of these 58% had had only one. A 2001 study proposed that improved contraceptive advice around the time of the abortion could substantially reduce repeat abortions, and so lower the overall rate. The authors reported, for example, that some providers were reluctant to provide a woman with an intra-uterine device (IUD) after an abortion on the grounds that it might interfere with the normal blood flow and they might not be able to determine whether the abortion was complete (Senlet et al. 2001). Two-thirds of the abortions in the country were carried out by private doctors and many of these were performed in their offices using predominantly curettage or menstrual regulation. Overall in Turkey between one-quarter and one-third of the abortions are carried out in Istanbul, despite the fact that it contains only just over 10% of the population (Senlet et al. 2001). We have seen in the Introduction that one of the reasons why abortion is relatively accepted is that Muslim religious scholars in the region predominantly believe abortion can be legal for the first 120 days of a pregnancy.

The high rates of repeat abortion led the Turkey Ministry of Health to initiate a pilot study into post-abortion family planning. This took place in the Zekai Tahir Burak Hospital. At the start of the study in 1991, 65% of women were given post-abortion contraception. The researchers instituted a four-part plan to increase uptake. These were, first, improved facilities and, second, improved staff attitudes. It showed, for example, that there were no extra risks with post-abortion IUD. Third, they gave accurate information about the wide range of abortion services and, finally, they improved the range of contraceptives on offer. They expanded the range to provide oral contraception, IUD, tubal ligation, vasectomy, implants and injectables. The take-up of contraception rose from 65% in 1991 to 97% in 1992. They then expanded the study in 1994 to include ten more hospitals, one of which dropped out. They found that six of the nine new hospitals increased their take-up of post-abortion contraception to over 90% and that there were significant changes in methods even in the first six months. IUD use more than doubled to 49% and tubal ligation increased to 15%. The abortion rate in Turkey has reduced. As several of its East European neighbours continue to have very high rates this led researchers to comment: 'The post-abortion program experience of Turkey can provide valuable lessons' (Senlet et al. 2001).

In the early 1990s an attempt was made to introduce medical abortion. However, mifepristone was not officially approved until 1994 and so the application was refused by the Commission at the Ministry of Health. At this point the Commission approved a study to gather data on medical abortion supported by the Population Council for terminating a pregnancy up to 56 days after last menstrual period. It aimed to test the efficacy of 200 mg mifepristone taken orally at the clinic and then two days later 400 mcg misoprostol taken orally either at home or at the clinic. During the study period 470 women were eligible and could choose either a medical or surgical abortion. There were 209 medical abortions and 149 surgical ones; the average length of pain was the same for both groups at between three and four days. Nine out of ten women having a medical abortion said that they would prefer it again compared with seven out of ten of those having a surgical abortion. The authors concluded that the findings supported the introduction of early medical abortion (Akin et al. 2005).

## Uzbekistan

The population was 27.3 million in 2006, the third most populous country from the fragmented Soviet Union. In 2003 the birth rate was 26 per thousand and the death rate was eight per thousand, a rate of natural increase of 1.8%. If current trends continue the population will grow to 38.7 million by the year 2050. However, the country has exhibited a declining family size. During the period 1985–1990 the total fertility rate was 4.4 children per woman (Population Division 2007c); in 1995–2000 it was 3.5, and in 2000–2005 it was 2.6. Family size has therefore declined by almost two children over a ten-year period. Life expectancy was 67 years in 2000–2005 (Wright 2006: 489). The country is 88% Muslim and most of these are Sunnis; 9% are Eastern Orthodox Christians and there are 3% believers of other religions. The capital is Tashkent, with a population of 2.1 million (Wright 2006: 700).

Until 1992, when it was part of the USSR, the country was known as the Uzbek Soviet Socialist Republic. Its law before independence followed the abortion law of the rest of the USSR in abortion being legalised a second time in 1955. The law currently allows abortion on request up to 12 weeks' gestation and up to 28 weeks on more restricted grounds. When it was part of the Soviet Union it had a relatively high abortion rate. In 1971 there were 156,000; in 1981 166,000 and they rose to a peak of 258,000 abortions in 1988, a rate of 61 per thousand women. By 1991 – the year before independence – it had reduced to 189,000, an abortion rate of 39 per thousand women aged 15–45 years. After independence the abortion rate began to fall. It declined to 23 per thousand in 1992 and by around half to 11.8 in 1996. The maternal mortality rates also showed evidence of this reduction declining from 38.9 per 100,000 births in 1988 to 10.5 in 1997 (Population Division 2007c).

Eighty-nine per cent of women knew of at least one contraceptive method and 40% were using a method which was provided free of charge. Of those using a method, 87% used the IUD. The abortion rate was relatively low and only 14% of pregnancies were terminated. There were two interesting findings from the study. One was that women in rural areas had an average of one birth more than women in urban areas: the total fertility rate was 3.7 children per mother in rural areas and 2.7 in urban ones. The second was that 96% of women breastfed for long periods. In all, 98% of those having abortions already had children (Digest 1998). In more recent years the abortion rate has fallen further year by year to 61,000 in the year 2000 and 51,000 in 2005; at this level the abortion rate per thousand women aged 15–45 is 7.2 and, although reporting may not be complete, it does seem that fertility in Uzbekistan is something of a success story and that women are having the number of children they desire (Johnston 2007d).

## Vietnam

The population in 2006 was estimated at 84.4 million and is expected to rise to 117.7 million by the year 2050. Over the years 2000–2005 the average woman had 2.2 children. The average length of life was 70 years, quite high for the region (Wright 2006: 489). Religions include Buddhism, Taoism, Roman Catholicism and indigenous religions but we do not have exact figures There was no written law allowing or prohibiting abortion in Vietnam between 1945 and 1962. In 1962, with the revision of the Law on Protection and Care of People's Health, abortion was made legal in the country. It seems the first year that official figures for the number of abortions were produced was 1978, when there were 70,281 reported. In 1987 the official level was reported at 811,176, rising to a peak of 1,380,000 in 1993. In the year 2000, 688,029 were reported, around a 50% reduction from the peak (Chinoy 2007; Johnston 2007e). In part this may have been because of a programme of action started in 1994 which campaigned for government and religious organisations to expand contraceptive facilities. During the 1990s the high levels of abortion translated into an average of 2.5 abortions during a woman's reproductive life. (Ganatra et al. 2004: 105).

The World Health Organization published a report in 1999 which revealed evidence that many women who thought they were having abortions were not in fact pregnant. It recommended that a history should be taken and a pelvic examination to establish pregnancy; if it could not be established, a urine test should be performed. The WHO report also recommended that facilities should not be paid on a fee-for-service basis as this was likely to encourage unnecessary operations. One problem to which the report also drew attention was that at the time of an abortion the opportunity to discuss future contraception was not taken to a marked degree; if this were changed the number of repeat abortions could be reduced (WHO 1999). Vietnam is one of the three countries with the highest abortion rates in the world, according to WHO. Every minute, 389 women become pregnant, 180 pregnancies being unplanned, and one woman dies from the complications of pregnancy (UN 2002).

IPPF makes the following comments about Vietnam:

> Young people contribute to more than 30% of the total number of abortion cases in Vietnam. This vulnerable group often comes from the rural areas and move to the cities to seek employment. Living stress, and peer pressure, together with poor knowledge on sexuality and family planning, lead them to risky sexual behavior and hence unwanted pregnancies. Often these young people, who are usually unmarried, seek abortion services when they are more than 24 weeks pregnant, and termination is then almost impossible. In Vietnam, only government hospitals are allowed to perform abortions, but many women go to private clinics for services, due to less visibility and protocols. Many of these private centers are not staffed with skilled providers and lack modern equipment, hence many women face complications following the procedure. However, even when abortion is legal, services are not easily accessible and often the cost is beyond the reach of those who need the service (personal communication).

IPPF further commented on the current situation that it was time for the government to energetically raise the abortion issue in the country and implement programmes to reduce abortion rates and human suffering.

## Yemen

The population was 21.4 million in 2006. In 2003 its birth rate was 43 per thousand and its death rate was nine per thousand, a rate of natural increase of 3.4%. It is expected that the population will almost quadruple to 84.4 million by the year 2050. During the period 2000–2005 the average woman had 6.0 children. This was a reduction from 7.7 in 1992 and 6.5 in 1997. In part this reduction might have been due to the National Population Strategy begun in 1991. Overall the reduction in fertility is slower than that in other Arab countries. One reason might be due to the tradition of early marriage: in 1985 the average age of marriage for girls was 13 years. The infant mortality rate in that year was 156, which means that the average woman had more than one child die before the age of 1 year (Al-Rabee 2003).

Life expectancy in 2000–2005 was 60 years, which was an improvement on 42 years in 1970 (Wright 2006: 483, 489). The country has substantial populations of both Shia and Sunni Muslims and small numbers of Jews, Christians and Hindus. The capital is Sana'a with a population of nearly 1 million. The population of Aden is 562,000 (Wright 2006: 704). It is a relatively poor country: for example, only 22% of births are attended by a skilled nurse or doctor. It also has high unemployment (UN 2003). North and South Yemen joined together on 22 May 1990 and this was followed by the growth in democracy and the establishment of political parties.

When contraception was developing in the country it was first practised mostly in the urban areas. In 1991–1992, 28% of married women in urban areas used modern methods of birth control compared with only 6% in the rural areas. In 2007 it was reported that only 10% of women aged 15–44 used modern methods of contraception (Population Division 2007d). A number of observers talk about the country having widespread abortion but we have not seen any local estimates as to numbers. The country has been receiving help from outside agencies. Marie Stopes International started work in the country in 1998 and has been providing services since that time. In February 2006 the British government promised 3 million pounds extra aid to help recover from the US gag rule.

A new development in March 2007 was the agreement made between the Abd-Kurin al-Archadi of the Ministry of Planning and International Co-operation and the UN Family Planning Association to set up a population reduction programme for the period 2007–2011. This entails improving contraception as well as other developments (United Press International 2007).

## Conclusion

The country analysis of Asia shows that women in the region make substantial use of abortion to control their fertility. It is clear that contraceptive services are underdeveloped in many countries. A more vigorous approach could reduce the number of abortions and improve women's health

# AFRICA

*I FAILED TO WITHDRAW BECAUSE I WAS
ENJOYING MYSELF. SHE CRIED THAT I HAD
IMPREGNATED HER. SHE THEN CHECKED THE
CALENDAR TO NOTE THE DATE AND TIME
THAT I HAD IMPREGNATED HER.*

Jagwe-Wadda et al. 2006

Africa has particular problems in the area of sexual health. The data for 2005 show that across sub-Saharan Africa 6.4% of adults have HIV, around 16 times the rate for Asia and over 12 times the rate for Latin America. Sub-Saharan Africa has a little over 10% of the world's population but 64% of the people living with AIDS. In 2005, worldwide the highest concentration of HIV/AIDS was the one in three (33.4%) in Swaziland. Botswana had a rate of 24.1%, Lesotho 23.2%, Zimbabwe 20.1%, South Africa 18.8% and Zambia 17.0% (Wright 2006: 491). Such a high incidence is having disastrous effects on the local population. Worldwide, since the first clinical evidence of HIV/AIDS in 1981, more than 65 million people have been infected with HIV and over 25 million people have died of AIDS. Estimates for 2005 gave a figure of 4.1 million people newly infected with HIV and 2.8 million deaths. Although unsafe abortion is not such a large problem as HIV/AIDS it is still an immense problem and one that may in part have similar solutions. Estimates for the year 2000 gave figures of 4.2 million unsafe abortions in Africa with a rate among women aged 15–44 of 24 per thousand. The number of deaths from unsafe abortion was estimated to be 29,800 with the UN estimating a case fatality of seven per thousand unsafe abortions (UN 2004: 89). This is the highest in the world and about seven times the rate for Latin America and the Caribbean (UN 2004: 89).

Africa's population growth has reduced in recent years. In the period 1970–1975 the fertility rate was an average of 6.7 children per woman. It fell to 5.6 in the period 1990–1995 and to 5.3 from 1995–2000 (UN 2004: 29).

IPPF provided the following information in 2007 (personal communication):

In almost all countries in the continent abortion laws are restrictive and modeled closely after the laws of the major colonial powers that governed them at independence. In all countries however, the law permits abortion for at least some indications such as to save the woman's life or to terminate a pregnancy resulting from rape or incest. Tragically even in countries with these legal exceptions safe abortion is rarely openly available, accessible or affordable. In general, political and religious leaders, policy makers, health professionals and communities are not aware of what the law permits. Women in general lack knowledge about their rights to abortion services for certain indications, yet every woman has a right to control her own sexuality, health and well being.

In Sub-Saharan Africa abortion is allowed by law without restrictions only in South Africa before twelve weeks of gestation and in Cape Verde before 14 weeks. In Mauritius about 50% of all pregnancies end up in induced but safe abortion since a majority of women can afford to pay for the services. The annual per capita income for that country is over US $8,000.

There have been some reviews of abortion laws in a few countries in the region over recent years which have resulted in the inclusion of additional grounds for which safe abortion can be provided. The latest is in Ethiopia where abortion may now be provided on request to all minors who may suffer physical or psychological trauma from an unwanted pregnancy (a minor in Ethiopia is anyone under 18 years of age).

One important development in Africa was the first ever regional conference on unsafe abortion in Addis Ababa in 2003. This brought together 112 people who included ministers of health, policy makers and media representatives. The conference called on governments to review restrictive laws and to provide increased funding for programmes which address unsafe abortion. The conference was co-convened by the African Partnership for Sexual and Reproductive Health and the Right of Women and Girls (Amanitare). The organisation's objectives include the promotion of bodily integrity and healthy reproduction, and the right to live free of coercion, violence or punishment related to sexuality or fertility (Hessini 2005: 91). Also in 2003 the African Union adopted a protocol on the rights of women in Africa. It called for states to protect women's rights by authorising abortion in the case of sexual assault, rape, incest and fetal impairment or where the pregnancy would endanger the mental or physical health of the woman (Hessini 2005: 92).

A first round in the liberalisation of laws occurred in the 1970s: Zambia (1972), South Africa and Namibia (1975), Liberia and Zimbabwe (1977). In the 1980s there were changes in the Seychelles (1981), Ghana (1985) and Cape Verde (1986). In the 1990s liberalisation occurred in Botswana (1991), Seychelles again (1994), Burkina Faso, South Africa again (1996) and in 2004 in Ethiopia. A movement to more restrictiveness occurred in Equatorial Guinea in 1991. Currently abortion is permitted on request in only three of 56 African countries: Cape Verde, South Africa and Tunisia (UN 2004: 88).

Regardless of the law, safe abortion services can be obtained by women with sufficient financial resources. In some countries only a few women are able to access these services while in others safe services are widely available. We will now consider the situation in the larger African countries. The United Nations geographical regions in Africa are as follows:

- **Eastern Africa** Burundi, Comoros, Djibouti, Eritrea, Ethiopia, Kenya, Madagascar, Malawi, Mauritius, Mozambique, Reunion, Rwanda, Somalia, Uganda, United Republic of Tanzania, Zambia, Zimbabwe
- **Middle Africa** Angola, Cameroon, Central African Republic, Chad, Congo, Democratic Republic of the Congo, Equatorial Guinea, Gabon
- **Northern Africa** Algeria, Egypt, Libya, Jamahiriya, Morocco, Sudan, Tunisia, Western Sahara
- **Southern Africa** Botswana, Lesotho, Namibia, South Africa, Swaziland
- **Western Africa** Benin, Burkina Faso, Cape Verde, Côte d'Ivoire, Gambia, Ghana, Guinea, Guinea-Bissau, Liberia, Mali, Mauritania, Niger, Nigeria, Senegal, Sierra Leone, Togo.

## Algeria

The population was estimated at 32.9 million in 2006 and the average woman had 2.5 children in 2005. Despite the civil war the life expectancy of the country had grown from 53 years in 1970 to 71 years in 2000 to 2005 and the infant mortality rate was 37 per thousand live births over this period (Wright 2006: 487). The population is 99% Sunni Muslim.

Algeria gained its independence from France on 5 July 1962. Its first free multi-party elections were held on 12 June 1990 and were won convincingly by the Islamic Salvation Front which received 188 seats out of 231. It was poised to take control of the government when the army seized power. The military's High Security Council postponed a return to democracy. Elections in June 1997 produced Algeria's first multi-party parliament since independence but the military remained in control and in a 'night of terror' in August 1967 Muslim fundamentalists killed over 300 people. One estimate is that civil strife and assassinations claimed the lives of 70,000 people between 1992 and 1998 (Chelala 1998). In April 1999 the army backed Abdelaziz Bouteflika who emerged as the only candidate for president; he reached an accord with the Islamic Salvation Front in return for an end to the uprising. Rebels who surrendered were offered an amnesty but after the period expired the military commenced a major offensive against the remaining rebels. By this time the groups had been organised as the 'Armed Islamic Group' (GIA). In 2004 Bouteflika was re-elected, winning a reported 84% of the vote (Wright 2006: 527).

The violence of the civil war had an important effect on abortion practice. According to the Algerian Criminal Code of 8 June 1966, abortion was legally allowed only to save the life of the woman. There were many cases of women becoming pregnant by rape. A meeting organised by the UN was told by Mrs Karadja that there was a so-called religious decree of certain fundamentalist groups in 1994 that 'wives of enemies were to be regarded as the spoils of war. Since then the kidnapping of women followed by rape had increased' (UN 1998). The British journal the Lancet reported that 1,600 women aged 13–20 had been kidnapped and raped by bands of armed Islamist groups. In addition at least 2,000 women had been raped and killed on the spot (Chelala 1998: 1413). There were few attempts to treat rape as a crime. Abdelhak Bererhi, an Algerian senator and former education minister said on French radio, 'It is indecent to compare rape in a police commissariat with a rape by a GIA terrorist' (UN 1998). This implies that rape by the police is not so unacceptable.

On 4 March 1998 the rape attacks led the Algerian government to ask the religious authorities to declare a fatwa allowing women raped in a political situation to have abortions. Four days later on International Women's Day, thousands of women demonstrated for a change in the law. This was agreed two months later (UN 1998).

In comparison with other African countries Algeria has relatively high contraceptive usage. It increased from 42% of married and cohabiting women in 1990 to 62% in the year 2000 and of these 60% were modern methods of contraception (UN 2004: 57).

## Burkina Faso

The population was estimated at 13.9 million in 2006. Over the period 2000–2005 life expectancy at birth was 47 years, an increase from 40 years in 1970. The population is 50% Muslim, 40% indigenous beliefs and 10% Christian. In the year 2003 the birth rate was 45 per thousand and the death rate 19 per thousand, a rate of natural increase of 2.6%. Infant mortality was 121 per thousand births during 2000–2005 (Wright 2006: 477). In 2005 the average woman had 6.5 children and for every thousand women there were 786 infant deaths. At current fertility and mortality rates the population will increase to 42.4 million by the year 2050 (Wright 2006: 48). The capital city is Ouagadougou with a population of 441,514 (1985 census).

Contraceptive use has not been common and in 1990 only 6% of women were using it. This increased slightly to 13% in 2000 (UN 2004: 5).

Abortion is legal only when the pregnancy presents risks to the mother's life, or in cases of rape, incest and fetal malformations. While a number of family planning needs remain unmet, constraints in accessing quality services often lead to unwanted pregnancies and illegal abortions, with unpredictable implications for the life of clients. A study by Rossier and colleagues (2004) used a new method of estimating the number of illegal abortions. They observed: 'People were not willing to talk of their own abortions but very willing to talk about those of others.' They accordingly set up a research programme in which they asked a random sample of the population in the capital who were in the fertile age range (15–49) about their friends and relatives with whom they had a close relationship. They sampled 963 women and 417 men of whom 44% named a confidant in the age range. They were informed about 163 illegal abortions which they calculated to represent a total rate of 1.1 abortions for the average woman during her lifetime. These were carried out by the woman herself in 26% of cases; six out of ten (61%) were carried out by a medically trained person such as a nurse; and around one in eight (13%) by a traditional healer. One-third of the abortions were by injection, one-fifth by dilation and curettage and one in eight by household drugs. The other third was not specified. Sometimes people had to make several attempts before the abortion was successful and Rossier and colleagues quote one man who said that first his girlfriend tried tablets but they were too bitter. He gave her money for roots but they also did not work. Consequently, he said:

> I took my girlfriend to another healer. I paid 6,000 FCFA (about $9) which I paid back afterwards. She told me she was feeling it was coming out, we were all glad and then nothing. I said if we did not hit hard things were going to become difficult. I explained the deal to my friend who repairs mopeds, who talked to other friends and his. They took him to Latfitenga. He scouted the place for me and two days later he and my girlfriend and I took off to have an injection in Latfitenga (Rossier 2004).

The injection achieved its purpose. From the figures of Ouagadougou, Rossier and colleagues calculated an abortion rate of 41 per thousand for women aged 15–49. For those aged 15–19 it was 61. Overall 60% of abortions resulted in complications and 14% of women needed treatment in a hospital. This research indicates the need to establish accessible curative health care systems.

## Cameroon

The population was estimated at 17.3 million in 2006. Over the period 2000–2005 life expectancy at birth was 49 years. The population is 40% indigenous beliefs (animist), 37% Roman Catholic and 20% Muslim. In the year 2003 the birth rate was 35 per thousand and the death rate 15 per thousand, a rate of natural increase of 2.0%. It is situated in Central Africa and has more than 230 ethnic groups and two official languages (English and French). Despite the ethnic diversity most Cameroonians have attached great importance to large families. In 2005 the average woman had 4.4 children and if trends continue the population will be 39.1 million by the year 2050 (Wright 2006: 481).

Contraceptive education in Cameroon is inadequate according to Schuster (2005) and helps explain why unwanted pregnancies occur. Contraceptive use increased from 15% of married and cohabiting women in 1990 to 20% in the year 2000. Of these 8% were modern methods of contraception (UN 2004: 57). Contraceptive use is therefore low and adolescents' access to education and information on sexual matters including contraception is largely restricted 'because of fear of encouraging immoral or unrestrained sexual behaviour' (Schuster 2005: 132). As far as married women are concerned evidence suggests a heavy reliance on the rhythm method. Gender roles enjoin women to be submissive. Women respondents 'used dubious methods such as drinking saltwater immediately after sexual intercourse' and even when they had access to modern contraception the risk of pregnancy was high because of their lack of knowledge about correct usage (Schuster 2005: 132).

Abortion is legal in Cameroon to save the health or life of the pregnant woman and in the case of rape. In addition there are well-equipped clinics which carry out abortions openly for women who can afford it. Clandestine abortions are carried out by a variety of people including trained midwives, so-called native doctors and lay abortionists. Prosecutions for illegal abortion are rare and women were more concerned about the public shaming that could occur if the abortion became widely known (Schuster 2005: 1301–32).

IPPF comments (personal communication):

Abortion is regarded by the general public as something that is widespread among 'girls/women of little virtue'. In some ethnic groups, girls who have children at an early age also are regarded as having little virtue. Hence, they resort to unsafe abortions as soon as an unwanted pregnancy occurs. The number of health establishments offering quality Family Planning services is increasing, but these are mainly concentrated in the large cities (Population Council 1998). There are problems related to the accessibility, availability and quality of emergency obstetrical care, as stated above. Only in the main hospitals is the treatment of incomplete abortion and surgical post-abortion care available (Republic du Cameroon 2001), and while in theory women can access legal abortion in the main hospitals and surgical in integrated health care centres, in practice the services are often inadequate (Ministere de la Sante Publique 2001). In 2000, an evaluation of emergency obstetric care in five zones showed that only 20 out of 487 institutions offered basic emergency obstetrical care and that only two offered complete emergency obstetrical care (Ministere de la Sante Publique 1999)

The law of 10th July 1980 is still valid and stipulates that only pharmacists can sell family planning drugs and methods, and only on prescription. However, in addition, a national official distribution system provides the methods to accredited health centres and NGOs. As far as abortion is concerned, the penal code considers it as infanticide and punishes both the woman who commits abortion and the person who helps in the act.

Even though society is becoming more and more conscious of the realities of the practice and consequences of illegal abortion, a law so strict does not allow wide public discussion. The abortion issue was not considered a priority during the 1999 National Symposium on Reproductive Health. Principles defined as 'ethical', have prevailed over practical and cause very serious public health considerations, to which field workers are confronted time and again (Republic De Cameroon 2002).

The legalisation of abortion in Cameroon has always been a contentious issue. Opinions are divided and there is a tendency to hide or ignore the reality of the high frequency of unsafe abortions. Abortion cases are usually undeclared. There have however, been isolated but dramatic cases denounced in newspapers articles, or by initiatives undertaken by NGOs working in the health sector or involved in Human Rights. The media reports cases of infanticide or child abandonment at least once a month, including cases of young girls who lose their lives after performing unsafe abortions by using unsound traditional methods.

In 1995 the number of unsafe abortions was estimated as 25–29 per thousand women aged 15–49 years, which had declined by 2000 to 20–25 per thousand women. Also in 2000 the estimated ratio of deaths due to unsafe abortion was relatively high at 90 per 100,000 live births. Schuster reports that on the gynaecology ward where she worked between November 1996 and October 1997 a total of 489 women were hospitalised; of these 107 (21.9%) were admitted for complications of an illegal abortion and eight of these died (2005: 135). She gave an example of an 18-year-old woman who had initially been admitted during the night with a diagnosis of malaria. The next day she was transferred to the gynaecology ward. She had a positive pregnancy test and a heavy vaginal discharge. Her notes read 'history not adequate, patient withholding information'. She died that afternoon before surgery could be performed. This example indicates that the woman's desire for secrecy conflicted with the provision of quality care.

Cameroon clearly has a need for better education, an improvement in services to the poorer groups who cannot afford good treatment, and a change in the law so that all can have safe legal treatment.

## Congo (formerly Zaire)

The population was estimated at 62.6 million in 2006. Over the period 2000–2005 life expectancy at birth was 52 years and has increased by only one year since 1970 (Wright 2006: 477). The population is 50% Roman Catholic, 20% Protestant, 10% Kimbanguist, 10% Muslim and 10% other (Wright 2006: 559). In the year 2003 the birth rate was 45 per thousand and the death rate 15 per thousand, a rate of natural increase of 3.0%. Infant mortality was 72 per thousand births during 2000–2005. In 2005 the average woman had 6.7 children and if trends continue the population will be 151.6 million by the year 2050 (Wright 2006: 482). The relatively high birth and infant mortality rate mean that for every thousand mothers 500 will suffer an infant death. The capital city is Kinshasa with a population of 2.7 million (1984 census).

Human Rights Watch (2005) said that women in Eastern Congo have suffered tremendous sexual violence. Victims have been from age 4 months to 84 years. There have been many cases of HIV/Aids due to rape which have not been diagnosed. One report said that before 1996 rape was usually carried out by a single 'admirer' and the results would often be marriage or there would be reparation by the payments of two or three goats to the victim. However, the war has resulted in many soldiers committing terrible acts of rape and mutilation of women. There are drugs which can protect against HIV/AIDS if taken up to 72 hours after an attack but few women take them. At the Panzi hospital in 1999, 290 women presented for treatment following rape or mutilation and this number increased to 1,289 in 2003. This is not necessarily due simply to an increase but also that women were more confident in travelling to the hospital. Observers report that 'social stigma has left large numbers of rape victims and children born of rape rejected by their families and communities' (Pratt and Werchick 2004). An unmarried girl who has been raped has little chance of marriage. If the pregnancy continues the baby is often rejected by the girl. One commented before the birth 'what if my baby looks like my rapist'. Pratt and Werchick report that one of the problems was that many soldiers believe that sex with a prepubescent or postmenopausal woman can give strength and protect from injury and death.

Abortion is legal only when the pregnancy threatens the woman's life or the fetus suffers from abnormalities. Clearly there is much to be done to achieve a peaceful environment where people can be safe and make their own choices about their lifestyle.

# Egypt

The population was estimated at 78.9 million in 2006. Over the period 2000–2005 life expectancy at birth was 69 years. The population is 94% Muslim (mostly Sunni) and 6% Coptic Christian (Wright 2006: 569). In the year 2003 the birth rate was 24 per thousand and the death rate five per thousand, a rate of natural increase of 1.9%. In 2005 the average woman had 3.1 children and if trends continue the population will be 127.4 million by the year 2050 (Wright 2006: 48).

Egypt was the first Arab country to adopt a national population policy. The government adopted a policy to reduce fertility in 1962 and established the Supreme Council for Population and Family Planning in 1965. In 1973, the responsibility for the delivery of family planning services was transferred to the Ministry of Health. Contraception is also available through a number of private sector agencies. In 1994 Cairo was the venue for the important International Conference on Population and Development. The Egyptian Family Planning Association, which developed from the National Population Commission, started providing reproductive health services countrywide in 1995. Contraceptive use increased from 41% married and cohabiting women in 1990 to 56% in the year 2000 and of these 54% were modern methods of contraception (UN 2004: 55). This is high usage in comparison with other countries in the area.

In 1995 a study was completed which led to improved post-abortion care. IPPF reported the following in March 2007 (personal communication):

> The IPPF Member Association currently has 139 clinics all over the country. The efforts of the Member Association to combat unsafe abortion have focused on encouraging men and women to use contraceptive methods in order to prevent unwanted pregnancies. In part this is by use of mobile clinics. The Member Association advocates combating unsafe abortion by maximizing access to quality family planning. A number of youth movements have been formed in the region including the Egyptian Association for Population and Development with some thousand members. This organization grew out of the 'friends of the forum' at the International Conference in Cairo.

> The Egyptian Member Association, which developed from the National Population Commission, has been providing reproductive health services country-wide since 1995. There has been a doubling in the use of modern contraceptives to over 54% in the twenty years until 2003. The Member Association clinics do not provide direct abortion services as, in Egypt, therapeutic abortion services cannot be provided in clinics. They therefore refer cases to the nearest hospitals.

> The Egyptian code of 1937 (sections 260–264) is still in place. It only allows abortion to save the life of the pregnant woman. However, it is sometimes interpreted as encompassing cases where the pregnancy may cause serious risks to the health of the pregnant woman or even in cases of fetal impairment. Public hospitals in Egypt receive approximately 336,000 cases of abortion per year. Using WHO classifications, 35% are spontaneous, 5% intended, and 60% represent probable intended abortion. Hemorrhage is the leading cause of maternal mortality and accounts for 38% of all maternal deaths.

In 1993 the maternal mortality ratio was 170 per 100,000 and 4.5% of maternal mortality was due to abortion (Maternal Mortality 2003) while in 2004 the maternal mortality ratio decreased to 84 per 100,000.

# Ethiopia

The population was estimated at 74.8 million in 2006. Over the period 2000–2005 life expectancy at birth was 48 years. The population is 45–50% Muslim, 35–40% Ethiopian Orthodox and 12% animist. In the year 2003 the birth rate was 40 per thousand and the death rate 20 per thousand, a rate of natural increase of 2%. In 2005 the average woman had 5.7 children and at current fertility and mortality rates the population will be 171 million by the year 2050 (Wright 2006: 486). The capital city is Addis Ababa (New Flower) with a population of 2.2 million (1993 estimate).

The health status and related indicators of the population of Ethiopia are among the worst in the world. Women of reproductive age and children up to the age of 15 constitute about 65% of the total population and are the most vulnerable groups.

Access to modern contraception is low. The IPPF local office reports that there is a 36% unmet need for family planning in the country, and that the contraceptive usage rate is estimated to be at 8%. A survey of unsafe abortion in selected health facilities in Ethiopia showed that the vast majority (87%) of women were aware of contraceptive methods, but only about half of the women ever used a method. Of those pregnancies that ended in abortion 60% were unplanned (personal communication).

Unsafe and illicit abortion often results from sexual violence such as rape and other harmful traditional practices. Maternal mortality is estimated to be 871 per 100,000 live births with 50% of the maternal deaths being due to unsafe abortions (Brookman Amissah and Moyo 2004). Besides high numbers of maternal deaths resulting from unsafe abortion, women also suffer from health problems that occur as a result of complications associated with pregnancy and childbirth. Most abortions were carried out under unhygienic or unsafe conditions, by unqualified personnel, including health assistants, anonymous persons or by the patients themselves. Methods used included plastic tubes, tree twigs, etc.

In 2002 a report from the Ministry of Health stated there is an urgent need for more information about safe abortion in order to plan effective programmes, policies and strategies to properly address the issue. 'No matter the provider's attitude on abortion, women need care and they need it immediately.'

In 2004 in order to reduce the harm caused by illegal abortion and to conform to international human rights treaties, Ethiopia expanded the circumstances under which abortion is permitted to include the pregnant woman's lack of capacity to care for a child because of her age or physical or mental health. Minors automatically fall under this provision. Prior to 2004 abortion was permitted only to save a woman's life or protect her physical health and in cases of rape, incest or serious fetal impairment. Ministry of Health guidelines now prescribe 'woman centered care', that is 'a comprehensive approach to providing abortion services that takes account the various factors that influence a woman's individual mental and physical health needs, her personal circumstances, and her ability to access services'. The guidelines also provide that abortions should be provided within three days of a woman's request, that proof of rape or incest is not required for abortions on those grounds, and that a minor is not required to present proof of age (Center for Reproductive Rights 2005).

# Kenya

The population was estimated at 34.7 million in 2006. Over the period 2000–2005 life expectancy at birth was 47 years. The population is 45% Protestant, 35% per Roman Catholic and 20% Muslim, indigenous beliefs and other. In the year 2003 the birth rate was 29 per thousand and the death rate 16 per thousand, a rate of natural increase of 1.3%. In the later 1960s and 1970s the average woman had over eight children. By 2005 the average woman had 5 children and if trends continue the population will be 44 million by the year 2050 (Wright 2006: 482). ) The capital city is Nairobi with a population of 1.3 million (1989 estimate).

In 1998 almost two in five (39.0%) married women of fertile age were using contraception. IPPF provided information about the situation in the country (personal communication).

In Kenya as in other parts of Africa, young people face severe threats to their health and general well-being. They are vulnerable to sexual assault and prostitution, early pregnancy and childbearing, unsafe abortion, malnutrition, female genital mutilation, infertility, and reproductive tract infections including sexually transmitted infections and HIV/AIDS. According to the 2003 Kenya Demographic and Health Survey, 44% of girls aged 15–19 years have had sexual intercourse and 19% are sexually active. Ninety four per cent of women in Kenya have heard of at least one modern contraceptive method, while 70% know of a traditional family planning method. Contraceptive prevalence rate is 39% with 32% of the currently married women using modern methods and 8% using traditional ones. Data suggests that approximately 308,000 abortions occur in the Kenya annually, with an estimated 20,300 women being hospitalized with abortion-related complications in public hospital. These lead to over 2,000 deaths annually which is a fatality rate of 10% (Brookman-Amissah and Moyo 2004).

According to the 2003 Kenya Demographic and Health Survey, maternal deaths represent 14% of all deaths of women aged 15–49 years. One third of these deaths were due to unsafe abortion. With a maternal mortality ratio of around 590 per 100,000 live births. Kenya has shown no signs of improving on this figure. Kenya like other countries has committed itself to reducing maternal mortality by 75% by the year 2015 in line with the Millennium Development Goals.

# Madagascar

The population was estimated at 18.6 million in 2006. Over the period 2000–2005 life expectancy at birth was 55 years. The population is 52% indigenous beliefs, 41% Christian and 7% Muslim (Wright 2006: 625). In the year 2003 the birth rate was 42 per thousand and the death rate 12 per thousand, a rate of natural increase of 3.0%. In 2005 the average woman had 5.2 children and if trends continue the population will be 46.3 million by the year 2050 (Wright 2006: 48).

In 1997 just one in five (19.4%) married and cohabiting women of fertile age were using contraception. This increased to just over one in five (21.0%) in the year 2000 (UN 2004: 57). Just over half of these (12%) were using modern methods of contraception.

# Morocco

The population was estimated at 33.2 million in 2006. Over the period 2000–2005 life expectancy at birth was 70 years. The population is just under 99% Muslim, 1% Christian and 0.2% Jewish (Wright 2006: 634). In the year 2003 the birth rate was 23 per thousand and the death rate six per thousand, a rate of natural increase of 1.7%. In 2005 the average woman had 2.7 children and if trends continue the population will be 47.1 million by the year 2050 (Wright 2006: 48).

A French law of 10 July 1939 prohibited the advertisement and sale of contraceptives. The government of Morocco has supported family planning since independence in 1956 and has recognised the influence of demographic factors. Contraceptives have been distributed free of charge in government family planning centres. Beginning with the development of the plan of 1968–1972, population issues, including family planning, have been accorded high priority in the planning process in Morocco. In 1971, the Association Marocaine de Planification Familiale, a private body, was established. Its role has evolved over the years, expanding its informational and educational activities to include clinical services. Family planning activities in Morocco have been fully integrated into the overall health care facilities, which have resulted in some financial difficulties and have hampered access to contraception by subsuming it under medical services. For these reasons, in the early 1980s, the government assigned to the Ministry of Public Health the responsibility for undertaking a policy of 'de-medicalisation' of family planning services in order to increase access to contraception. In addition, two innovative programmes were introduced, one involving mobile clinics providing maternal and child health and family planning services in remote rural areas, and the other involving systematic home visits to encourage the use of contraception and to provide family planning and primary health care services.

Contraceptive use increased from two in five (39%) married and cohabiting women in 1990 to two-thirds (65%) in the year 2000 and of these 54% were modern methods of contraception (UN 2004: 57). Morocco's abortion law was first liberalised in 1967. At that time, Article 453 of the Penal Code was amended by Royal Decree (1 July) to provide that the performance of an abortion would not be punished when it was a necessary measure to safeguard the physical health of the woman and was openly performed by a physician or a surgeon with the consent of the spouse. If there is no husband or the husband refuses or is prevented from giving his consent, the physician or surgeon may not perform the abortion without the written opinion of the chief medical officer of the province or prefecture, certifying that the intervention is the only means of safeguarding the health of the woman. If the physician believes that the woman's life is in jeopardy, the consent of the spouse or opinion of the chief medical officer is not required. The physician or surgeon must, however, give his opinion to the chief medical officer of the province or prefecture.

In all other cases, abortion is illegal under the Penal Code, although some evidence exists that fetal impairment may be taken into account under medical indications. Any person performing an illegal abortion is subject to one to five years' imprisonment and payment of a fine of 120–500 Moroccan dirhams. The penalty of imprisonment is doubled in the case of persons who regularly perform abortions. Medical and health personnel who perform an illegal abortion are subject to the same penalties, as well as to temporary or permanent suspension from practising their profession. A woman who induces her own abortion or consents to it being induced is subject to six months' to two years' imprisonment and payment of a fine of 120–500 dirhams. Local IPPF commentators suggest (personal communication) that despite the law illegal abortion appears to be widespread in Morocco, with many women resorting to it as a contraceptive method. It appears that the incidence of illegal abortion is underestimated. Many women obtaining an illegal abortion appear to be married women from the urban upper and middle classes who undergo one in a private clinic. Surveys of public hospitals suggest that a significant number of admissions are of women from the lower socio-economic groups suffering from complications of septic abortion.

## Mozambique

The population was estimated at 19.7 million in 2006. Over the period 2000–2005 life expectancy at birth was 42 years. The population is 50% indigenous beliefs, 30% Christian and 20% Muslim. In the year 2003 the birth rate was 37 per thousand and the death rate 23 per thousand, a rate of natural increase of 1.4%. In 2005 the average woman had 5.3 children and if trends continue the population will be 31.3 million by the year 2050 (Wright 2006: 483). The country has suffered from years of civil war which, together with poverty, has led to poor overall health care. The capital city is Maputo with a population of 1.0 Million (1987 estimate).

Contraceptive use is low. The United Nations stated in 1999 that it was used by 7.3% (UN 2004). An article based on 2002 data showed that it was used by only 5% of married women. Abortion has a quasi-legal status. Although strictly allowed only for the woman's life or health a 1981 Ministry of Health decree supported a broad interpretation of this risk. Consequently abortion on request has been available in several public hospitals ever since (Gallo et al. 2004). Most of these abortions are performed by using misoprostol followed by manual vacuum aspiration 24 hours later. The cost of an abortion in 2002 was about USD 15 which is a substantial sum in a country where 78% of the population were known to live on less than $2 a day.

The maternal mortality rate was estimated in 2002 at 1,000 deaths per 100,000 deliveries, one of the highest rates in the world. According to Gallo et al., one in seven women die during pregnancy (2004). These deaths are in large part related to unsafe abortions and in 1995 a study conducted in Maputo Central Hospital (Gallo et al. 2003) found that women attending for complications tended to be the younger and poorer women. Four out of five said that they did not know of the possibility of hospital-based abortions. Others had difficulty with the large amount of information needed by hospitals and data from a 'responsible male'.

In 2002 the Ministry of Health conducted an assessment of abortion services to inform efforts to make abortion safer. The study surveyed 461 women in 37 public hospitals and four health centres which encountered abortion-related complications. In addition 128 providers were interviewed. The results showed that the patients had endured a lengthy waiting time for treatment. Fewer women were receiving pain relief than providers thought were usual and less than half the women received follow-up care information. Of those women who wanted to avoid pregnancy only 27% said that they had received contraceptive advice. The results of the survey led to the Ministry's efforts to improve training of providers (Gallo et al. 2004).

# Nigeria

The population in 2006 was estimated at 131.8 million in 2006 but is predicted to almost double to 258 million in 2050. In the period 2000–2005 the average woman had 5.6 children and life expectancy at birth was only 43 years. This is a reduction from 44 in 1970. The infant mortality rate was 114 per thousand births (Wright 2006: 488). In 2003 the rate of increase in the population was 2.5%. The religion is 50% Muslim, 40% Christian and 10% indigenous beliefs. Although Lagos, with 13.4 million people, is the largest city, the capital is Abuja with a population of 306,000 (Wright 2006: 642). In 1990 less than one in 17 (6%) married or cohabiting women were using contraception. This increased to one in six (16%) in the year 2000 and over half these were using modern methods (UN 2004: 57).

In 1996–1997 Henshaw and colleagues estimated that there were 610,000 abortions in Nigeria each year, a rate of 25 per thousand women aged 15–44, which is comparable to that of the United States (Henshaw et al. 1998). This is higher than a 1980 estimate of a government committee of inquiry of 500,000 illegal abortions (Population Division 2007e). This survey, which was based on a study of 672 facilities, found that 27% of private physicians and 15% of public facilities performed abortions about equally by dilation and curettage and manual vacuum aspiration. The abortion rate was lower in the poorer north of the country (10 per thousand women aged 15–44 in the north-west and 13 in the north-east) and higher in the south where there was more wealth (32 in the south-east and 46 in the south-west, where Lagos is situated). With so many providers available, abortions can be obtained from physicians at a modest cost that often ranges around $10–$15, but many women prefer the convenience, privacy and lower cost of non-physicians or chemists.

These abortions are carried out despite the fact that they are largely illegal. Two laws apply to the country. In the largely Muslim north the law is the Penal Code of 1959, while in the south the Criminal Code of 1916 is in effect. This second law is based on the British 1861 act, which has been interpreted liberally in at least one case along the lines of the British 1938 Bourne decision to include wider grounds, including rape (see pp.36–7).

The high levels of unsafe abortion mean that it is the major cause of mortality for women under the age of 20. A study carried out from 1992–1994 in Ilorin found that 53% of those in hospital for the complications of abortion were aged 15–19 (Brookman Amissah and Moyo 2004). Overall one in three maternal deaths is due to abortion, which is much higher than the one in eight for West Africa (Phillips 1999). Part of the reason for the high death rate may be the fact that an estimated 26% of women with complications do not seek medical help (Grimes et al. 2006). One such death was that of Gloria Oguntola who bled to death and whose father, John, was quoted as saying, 'We do not know who to hold responsible because she could not tell us before she died' (Olori 2007). Other women suffer long-term health consequences. Toyin Aje became pregnant but her boyfriend told her he would not help bring the baby up. She sought an abortion but was unable to get one in a public hospital. She sought help from a man who worked in a pharmacy in the Abuja. He was neither a doctor nor a pharmacist but sold her drugs. She was five months pregnant and the fetus died and was retained in her uterus. She began to experience severe pain and was eventually treated in hospital. Although they were able to save her life she was told that she would be sterile (Olori

2007). Such incidents are common and overall only 40% of Nigerian abortions are estimated as being carried out by doctors.

In 1982 an attempt to liberalise the law was sponsored by the Society of Gynecologists and Obstetricians of Nigeria. This would have allowed abortion on the grounds that two physicians agreed 'there were substantial risks to the life of a pregnant woman, or injury to her physical and mental health or to any existing children in her family greater than if the pregnancy were terminated'. There would have been exceptions for conscience and the potential law bears strong overtones of the debate at the time of the British 1967 act. The change was opposed by religious groups and by the Nigerian National Council of Women's Societies and failed (Population Division 2007e).

The government showed its concern about overpopulation when in 1988 it instituted a national population policy which encourages family planning, but progress toward modern forms of contraception has been slower than most would like.

The case for a new law and more liberal practice remains strong. In 1991 the Federal Ministry of Health called for a change in the law (Henshaw et al. 1998). Boniface Oye-Adenirian the president of the African Medical Association and an obstetrician and gynaecologist in Lagos commented:

> For us to reduce the carnage to our women through unsafe abortions, the law has to regulate abortion services, determine who performs it and where it can be performed. If abortion services become more available in public hospitals quacks will be discouraged (International Press News 2007).

There is a strong case for increasing the availability of safe operations.

## South Africa

The population was estimated at 44.2 million in 2006. Over the period 2000–2005 life expectancy at birth was 49 years. The population is 68% Christian, 29% traditional beliefs and 3.5% Muslim and Hindu. In the year 2003 the birth rate was 19 per thousand and the death rate 18 per thousand, a rate of natural increase of 0.1%. In 2005 the average woman had 2.7 children and at current fertility and mortality rates the population will decline to 40.2 million by the year 2050 (Wright 2006: 483). Contraceptive use increased from half (51%) of married and cohabiting women in 1990 to 58% in the year 2000 and nearly all of these were modern methods of contraception (UN 2004: 57).

The earlier policies on abortion were in part associated with apartheid. Before 1975 abortion could be carried out under common law if there was a threat to 'a woman's well being'. The white political leadership was concerned that population changes were adverse to it. The Minister of Bantu Administration and Development, MC Botha, asked whites to have more children to ensure continued existence as a Christian and Western country on the continent of Africa. Women were given tax advantages to encourage them to have children. In contrast there were attempts to encourage the black population to use family planning. Consequently birth control became associated by some people with maintaining the apartheid regime. The Abortion and Sterilization Act was introduced in 1975 to restrict abortion. It allowed it only on the grounds of physical and mental health, sexual crimes such as rape and incest, and fetal abnormality. The bureaucracy for obtaining an abortion was immense. For example, the approval of two physicians was needed and neither of these was to be the one to perform the operation. Consequently there were few abortions carried out – around a thousand a year under the act (Guttmacher et al. 1998). Rich women could often obtain abortions by doctors performing a dilatation and curettage in their office; this was risky for them as it was illegal. Other rich women could fly to London and many did so. Poor women were reportedly using knitting needles or detergents or attending illegal and often unskilled practitioners (Guttmacher et al. 1998). In the period 1975–1996 there were an estimated 120,000 to 250,000 abortions a year. In 1994 the South African Medical Research Council carried out a study and found there were 45,000 hospital admissions and that over 400 women had died. The cost of the hospitalisation of women was calculated at $4.4 million (personal communication).

The introduction of democracy led to a new abortion law as the African National Congress (ANC) supported it and it was part of its programme in the 1994 elections. The relevant statement was: 'Every woman must have the right to choose whether or not to have an early termination according to her own beliefs.' The law was passed by 209 votes to 87 on 11 December 1996 and came into effect on 1 February 1997. It granted abortion on request in the first 12 weeks of pregnancy; one commentator said that the law aimed to grant universal access to services for all women by giving them the sole right of consent. It also provided for nurse-midwives to carry out abortions (Hessini 2005). From 13–20 weeks' gestation abortion was to be allowed on more restricted grounds. It was permitted 'if a medical practitioner believes that the pregnancy threatens the mental or physical health of the woman or fetus' or in the case of rape and incest, or if it 'affects the woman's socio-economic situation'. After 20 weeks, abortion could be carried out in the case of severe fetal abnormality or in the case of threat to the woman's life or health. The law was passed despite strong opposition from certain religious factions but with the support of women's groups and other health campaigners. One singular feature of the law is that it permits abortion by nurse-midwives who are trained and certified. Many abortions are now performed by nurses.

Legal abortion was a little slow to take effect because of the reluctance of hospitals to provide the service and the small number of non-hospital providers. In 1997 there were only 34,000 recorded and in 1998, 50,000. These figures were well below the estimates for the number of illegal abortions before the act. The numbers then rose only slightly and were 59,000 in 2000. They then began to rise more substantially to 90,000 in 2003 and 114,000 in 2004 (Johnston 2005).

## Sudan

The population was estimated at 41.2 million in 2006. Over the period 2000–2005 life expectancy at birth was 56 years. The population is 70% Sunni Muslim, 25% indigenous beliefs and 5% Christian (mainly in the south). In the year 2003 the birth rate was 36 per thousand and the death rate 10 per thousand, a rate of natural increase of 2.6%. In 2005 the average woman had 4.2 children and if trends continue the population will be 60.1 million by the year 2050 (Wright 2006: 678). The capital City is Khartoum with a population of 925,000 (1993 census).

In 1983 the government attempted to institute Islamic law throughout the country. This led to riots throughout the south and in the following year a state of emergency. Sudan supported Iraq's invasion of Kuwait in 1991 and in 1995 the UN endorsed an accusation that the country was sheltering the Islamic militants who attempted to assassinate the Egyptian president, Hosni Mubarak. In 1998 the USA launched cruise missiles at Khartoum to retaliate for the bombing of its embassies in Tanzania and Kenya and to destroy what it claimed was a chemical weapons factory (Wright 2006: 678–9). The country has also been torn by civil war in the south and west during which many women have been raped. This led to Fetter commenting: 'Violence is systematically used as a weapon of war by the Janjaweed – a gross breach of international humanitarian law.' She continues to maintain that around one in 20 women suffering rape become pregnant but that this is not the only possible problem. Women may also be rejected by their husbands or suffer pelvic inflammatory disease or HIV infection. The law in the Sudan does allow abortion to save the life of the woman and for rape if it is requested by the woman not more than 90 days after the offence occurred (Fetter 2006). Research published in 1999 stated that abortion was common in Western Dinka, which is in south-west Sudan (personal communication).

Contraceptive use has been low and, for example, in north Sudan only used by one in ten (9%) of married women in the year 2000 (UN 2004: 57).

# Tanzania

The population was estimated at 37.4 million in 2006. Over the period 2000–2005 life expectancy at birth was 46 years. The population is 35% Muslim, 35% indigenous beliefs and 30% Christian. In the year 2003 the birth rate was 40 per thousand and the death rate 17 per thousand, a rate of natural increase of 2.3%. This rate of increase has reduced from 3.2% during 1990–1995 (Population Division 2007f). In 2005 the average woman had 4.7 children and if trends continue the population will be 69.1 million by the year 2050 (Wright 2006: 483). The capital City is Dar es Salaam with a population of 1.1 million (Wright 2006: 686).

Tanzania is a very poor country; Dr Lucy Nkya reported that two sex workers were actually physically fighting over a used condom. They wanted to clean and reuse it (Mohagheghpour 1997).

The economy took a downturn in the 1990s owing to a number of factors including the debt problem, Rwandan refugees and general economic malaise. This led to a worsening of sexual and reproductive health for women. The country has a relatively high incidence of HIV/AIDS and in 2005 results showed 7.6% of men and 9.9% of women were infected with the virus (MSI 2007b).

In 1959 the Family Planning Association of Tanzania was established in Dar es Salaam. It came to be known as UMATI and grew to have national coverage. It said that it was going to concentrate on providing help to parents. This approach aimed to refute some of the criticism that promoting contraception would encourage promiscuity amongst the young. In 1969 the family planning groups affiliated to the International Planned Parenthood Federation and in 1974 the government became involved and integrated family planning with maternal and child health. The development of contraceptive services led to an increase in the percentage of women using modern methods from 10.4% in 1991 to 25.4% in 1999. In the 1990s the high rate of breastfeeding helped keep the pregnancy and abortion rate down and in 1991–2000 the median length of breastfeeding was 21 months (Mturi and Hinde 2001). The 2005 figures indicate there is still a need for more contraception as over one in five (21.8%) married women suffered an unmet need (Lusiola 2005).

The abortion law in Tanzania derives from the 1861 British law together with the liberalisation of the 1938 Bourne judgment and subsequent developments which allow the protection of the physical or mental health of the woman (Francome 1984a). As this law is relatively restrictive there are many unsafe abortions. In Tanzania in 1993 the cost per day of post-abortion care was over seven times the annual amount allowed by the Ministry of Health for per capita health expenses (Brookman Amissah and Moyo 2004). A 1987 study in Dar es Salaam surveyed 300 women who were in hospital after early pregnancy loss. It found that 31% had had an induced abortion (Population Division 2007). A study published in 1999 found that in Tanzania one-third of the victims of unsafe abortion were teenagers and that of these almost half were 17 years or younger. Safe operations are expensive to purchase in Tanzania and so can usually only be purchased by older women who have greater resources (Mundigo and Indriso 1999). An innovative study was into the role of the male partners at the time of the abortion. In 2005 it reported that of 213 men accompanying their partners, 44% of single men and 81% of married men had used birth control. In part this will have been due to age and, though the figures are relatively small it does suggest a need to spread contraceptive information to the unmarried. This study also proposed that there was a need for men to be more involved in post-abortion counselling in the hope that contraception usage will be increased and the abortion rate reduced (Rasch and Lyaruu 2005).

Marie Stopes Tanzania (MST) provides 30% of the family planning activities in Tanzania and 80% of the sterilisations. In 2001 the US foreign aid policy reinstituted a ban on grants to organisations involved with abortions. Marie Stopes Tanzania defied Bush and refused to stop providing abortions to those who qualified under the law. This did, however, lead to the organisation having to lay off 13% of its staff.

## Togo

The population was estimated at 5.5 million in 2006. Over the period 2000–2005 life expectancy at birth was 54 years. The population is 51% indigenous beliefs, 29% Christian and 20% Muslim. In the year 2003 the birth rate was 35 per thousand and the death rate 12 per thousand, a rate of natural increase of 2.3%. In 2005 the average woman had 5.1 children and if trends continue the population will be 10 million by the year 2050 (Wright 2006: 48). The 1998 demographic and health survey, the most recent in Togo, shows that just under one in four (23.5%) married women were using contraception and that of these only 7% were using modern methods (UN 2004: 64). This figure rose to 10% in 2003 (Ministére de la Sante 2003).

Induced abortion is still a criminal act in Togo, punishable under a law based on the French 1920 act banning incitement to commit an abortion and anti-conception propaganda. In 1981, the government promulgated a new penal code which was based on the law of 1920, with a few minor modifications. The current situation is that abortion is legal in the first three months of pregnancy only if the life of the woman is in danger or if the pregnancy is the result of rape or incest. The decision to terminate the pregnancy is taken by a panel of three doctors. These limited provisions concern only a limited number of cases and so do not substantially reduced illegal abortion rates.

There are no national data about the number of induced abortions and authorities seem hostile to any liberalisation or decriminalisation of abortion. They have often denied the existence of the problem and therefore ignored it. This is because of traditional ways of thinking and the severe condemnation of abortion on the part of the religious authorities. The data that exist are taken from hospital statistics and medical studies concerned with the complications of abortion or from studies of young people. The hospital statistics reveal that a large proportion of maternal mortality is the result of induced abortion. At the university hospital in Lomé, a study of 191 maternal deaths in 1991 showed that in 32% of these deaths the initial cause was an induced abortion (Toussa-Ahossu 1991). In 1996, a study carried out in the Central and Maritime regions with a sample of 1,854 schoolgirls (in their last five years at school), showed that 23% had already been pregnant, that 86% of these pregnancies were ended by an induced abortion and that 8% of cases ended with the removal of the uterus because of complications (KL Adognon unpublished paper).

A 1996 study on the prevalence of pregnancy among students in Togo aged from 12 to 26 showed that 84% of these pregnancies ended in induced abortion. According to other studies involving female clients of family planning centres and pupils, 24% of the female clients and 23% of the pupils said that they had had at least one abortion (Amergee 1999). Finally, a study in 2001 involving 3,459 women, from all over Togo, observed that 9% said that they had had at least one abortion (19% in Lomé), but this figure seems low in comparison with other information (Unite de Recherche Demographic 2002).

State hospitals as well as religious and private hospitals treat the complications produced by induced abortions. Curettage has been the method mainly used but vacuum aspiration has begun to be used too (for example, at the university hospital in Lomé). The providers are gynaecologists and general practitioners, medical assistants and occasionally nurses. These groups also offer abortion in certain medical practices and private clinics but they remain illegal.

At present, no single-issue organisations are campaigning openly in favour of abortion. However, there is a joint activity of the government (Ministry of Social Action) and a civil society (Group for Reflection and Action, Women Democracy and Development and Women in Law and Development in Africa) for a general improvement in the legislation relating to sexual and reproductive health, and, in particular, the repeal of the law of 1920 and the development of a family code more favourable to the condition and rights of women.

## Tunisia

The population was estimated at 10.2 million in 2006. Over the period 2000–2005 life expectancy at birth was 73 years. The population is 98% Muslim, 1% Christian and 1% Jewish and other religions (Wright 2006: 690). In the year 2003 the birth rate was 17 per thousand and the death rate 5 per thousand, a rate of natural increase of 1.2%; this is below half the rate of increase in 1985 which was 2.6%. The Tunisian government has achieved significant results, with the total fertility rate decreasing from 7.2 children per woman in 1965 to 3.4 in 1991, 2.6 in 2000 and in 2005 the average woman had 1.9 children. If trends continue the population will be 12.9 million by the year 2050 (Wright 2006: 48). The capital is Tunis with a population of 674,000.

Contraceptive use is high. It increased from 53% of married and cohabiting women in 1990 to 70% in the year 2000 (UN 2004: 57). In 1965 Tunisia became the first Muslim country to liberalise its abortion law. The Tunisian Penal Code of 1913 and the legislative decrees of 1920 and 1940, which amended the abortion provisions of the code, had all prohibited abortion except to save the life of the pregnant woman. A law of 1 July 1965 amended the code to allow abortion to be performed during the first three months of pregnancy, if a couple had at least five living children, and at any time during pregnancy if the continuance of pregnancy posed a danger to the health of the pregnant woman. This law was regarded by many as being far too restrictive and so a more liberal one was passed. Tunisia's current abortion law dates from 1973 and it authorises abortions on request during the first three months of pregnancy. After this period an abortion may be performed when there is a risk to the physical or mental health of the mother or that the unborn child will suffer from a serious disease or infirmity. The performance of abortion is subsidised by the government in the same way as all other medical services and those entitled to receive free health care can obtain an abortion free of charge in public hospitals.

The liberalisation of abortion was part of a national policy directed at reducing fertility as a means of improving economic development. In 1973, when the new abortion law was approved, the Office Nationale de la Famille et de la Population was created to direct the family planning programme. Subsequently in 1988 legislative action was complemented by other measures intended to raise the status of women and decrease fertility. The country began providing schooling for both sexes and supported the right of women to practise contraception. It also used the media to encourage family planning which was fully integrated into the basic health care system, and specialised (maternal health) wards were created to provide abortions and other services.

IPPF reports (March 2007 personal communication) that most recent data show the average Tunisian user of family planning to be aged 30 years, have 3.7 living children and to have been married nine years. Although high parity is no longer a requirement to obtain an abortion, the majority of women already have four or more children when they seek one. The 1996 rate of 8.6 abortions per thousand women aged 15–44 is remarkably low for a developing country, although official statistics omit legal abortions performed in the private sector. The true rate is estimated to be around 11 per thousand women aged 15–44 which is still very low considering the family planning programme. Despite the success of the national family planning programme, contraceptive users enter the programme at a relatively advanced age, indicating that contraception and abortion are used mainly to prevent subsequent births once the desired number of children has been reached.

## Uganda

The population was estimated to be 28.2 million in 2006. Over the period 2000–2005 life expectancy at birth was 47 years. The population is 33% Roman Catholic, 33% Protestant, 16% Muslim and 18% indigenous beliefs (Wright 2006: 693). In the year 2003 the birth rate was 47 per thousand and the death rate 17 per thousand, a rate of natural increase of 3.0%. In 2005 the average woman had 7.1 children and if trends continue the population will increase to 103.2 million by the year 2050 (Wright 2006: 483). Its infant mortality rate in 2000–2005 was 81 per thousand births. The country is very poor with there being only one doctor for over 18,000 people (Jagwe-Wadda et al. 2006). The capital city is Kampala with a population of 773,000 (1991 census).

In 1995 a survey showed that only one in seven (14.8%) women were using contraception. This increased to nearly one in four (23%) in the year 2000 and around half these were using modern methods (UN 2004: 57). This will have increased especially due to the concern with HIV/AIDS. Uganda's population growth is the third highest in the world and in 2004 it had a condom shortage. MSI Uganda was contracted by the UK's Department for International Development to provide an emergency supply of 20 million condoms. This they did and continued to develop 'Life Guard Pink' funded by the Global Fund to fight AIDS, tuberculosis and Malaria. This development has provided condoms which even the poorest user groups could afford. In 2007, MSI Uganda reported it planned to distribute over 225 million Life Guard condoms over the next five years. Overall Ugandans use over eleven million condoms each month (MSI 2007c).

Abortion is illegal except to save the life of the woman. Unsafe abortion is common with one estimate placing the figure at 300,000 a year for women aged 15–49. This provides an overall abortion rate of 54 per thousand. Abortion is seen as shameful within the society and consequently women hide the fact that they have had one. Despite this, a study of 40 *bodabodamen* (motor cycle taxi drivers) found that almost half their partners had had an abortion. A 40-year-old man told how he came to make his girlfriend pregnant and to her having an abortion:

> I went to her place and asked her for sex. She refused claiming she was not in her safe period. I was burning with passion so I convinced her that I was going to time [my ejaculation]. I failed to withdraw because I was enjoying myself. She cried that I had impregnated her. She then checked the calendar to note the date and time that I had impregnated her. And that is what happened exactly (Jagwe-Wadda et al. 2006).

It is estimated that 20% of women with complications from unsafe abortion do not seek treatment (Grimes et al. 2006). This may be one of the reasons that one-third of maternal deaths are due to unsafe abortion (Religious Tolerance 2005). Overall it is estimated that 85,000 women are taken to hospital each year with the after-effects of unsafe abortion (Jagwe-Wadda et al. 2006). The difficulties faced can be gauged by a study in Mulago Hospital, Kampala from 1983–1987. This found that the main adverse effects were sepsis, haemorrhage and genital tract trauma. In 1993 a study in Kampala found that one in five maternal deaths was due to abortion. However, some women have minimal problems – a young woman told how she visited the abortionist: 'She boiled the herbs and gave me a bottle to drink, and the pregnancy stopped. The pregnancy was still young and so the drug given was not so strong.' Others' experiences are much worse and when a 40-year-old urban male was asked why women did not seek help when they had post-abortion problems he stated:

> It is because of ignorance. When the fetus comes out they do not get to know what remains inside. The daughter of a friend of mine died under similar circumstances. She fell very sick after stopping a pregnancy and she never sought treatment. By the time her father realized it and decided to take her for treatment it was too late and she died (Jagwe-Wadda et al. 2006).

There are social changes occurring, particularly the increased provision of condoms. The 2000 Demographic and Health survey showed that amongst women 15–49 years 38% of pregnancies were unplanned (Jagwe Wadda et al 2006). If this percentage can be reduced by improved use of condoms and other contraceptives then the population increase could be reduced to more manageable proportions.

## Zambia

The population was estimated at 11.5 million in 2006. Over the period 2000–2005 life expectancy at birth was 37 years, a reduction of ten years since 1970. The population is 50–75% Christian, 24–49% Muslim and Hindu, and 1% traditional beliefs. In the year

2003 the birth rate was 40 per thousand and the death rate 24 per thousand, a rate of natural increase of 1.6%. In 2005 the average woman had 5.4 children and if trends continue the population will be 18.5 million by the year 2050 (Wright 2006: 48). The capital city is Lusaka with a population of 982,000 according to the 1990 census (Wright 2006: 705). One-fifth of Zambia's population is infected with the HIV virus.

Contraceptive use increased from one in ten married and cohabiting women in 1990 to nearly one in four (23%) in the year 2000 and nearly all of these used modern methods of contraception (UN 2004: 57).

Abortion in Zambia is based on the 1972 act which follows the wording of the British law: 'Abortion is allowed when the continuance of the pregnancy would involve risk to the life of the pregnant woman greater than if the pregnancy were terminated.' Fred de Sam Lazaro comments (2004) on the abortion law: 'Abortion is legal in Zambia but in practice it is difficult to obtain one. The women must first consult with one doctor and then get the approval of three other physicians before going to one of the few facilities.' Dr F Chanda, a gynaecologist at one of Lasaka's main hospitals, stated that dozens seek abortions each day but that very few have the legal referrals and furthermore many were suffering from illegal abortions. He continued to state that there were problems because 'some women don't know where they can have a safe abortion' (Population Division 2007g). A 15-year-old with the pseudonym Agnes and pregnant by her boyfriend was described in a newspaper:

> She thought about her parents, they were strict and she thought about what people would think of her. She went to see a retired nurse in one of the compounds. The nurse said she could perform the abortion at a fee, which she agreed to. According to Agnes the abortion was carried out and it was painful. She said the abortion still haunts her because she believes she committed a sin (Chakwe 2007).

Planned Parenthood of Zambia is popular amongst the village women and one commentator states: 'The average woman has six children. It makes it easy to understand why women in the valleys of Naluyanda celebrated the arrival of Justin Kapila the contraceptive man.' He continued to say that 'safe medical services are even more rare in Zambia's vast rural areas' (de Sam Lazaro 2004).

Some Christian groups propose abstinence as an alternative to the use of condoms and modern family planning methods to prevent unwanted pregnancies and HIV. For example Bishop Banda was quoted: 'We can increase young people's ability to postpone sexual involvement until they are married' (Religion and Ethics 2004). This abstinence approach is one put forward by the US Right as part of a solution to the HIV/AIDS epidemic in the country. The gag rule instituted by the Republicans in 2001 prohibiting funds for groups involved with abortion has prevented a comprehensive approach. The Planned Parenthood Federation of Zambia felt it had to stand firm on the issue and its lack of funds led to its being obliged to lay off 26 of its 68 staff (Religion and Ethics 2004).

The US funds for HIV/AIDS increased six times under the Republicans but the overall aid for family planning has started small and decreased. However, the country has received funds from the Japan International Co-operation Agency (Population Division 2007g).

There was a large march for women's rights in Washington DC on 9 May 2004 at which Hilary Fyfe of Zambia stated: 'Women no longer have choices and those who need information cannot get it.' In Zambia abortion is legal but four doctors and the woman's husband must endorse the woman's decision. 'By then it is too late and so we have a lot of unsafe abortions, teenager pregnancies and baby dumping' (Cliff 2004).

## Zimbabwe

The population was estimated at 12.2 million in 2006. Over the period 2000–2005 life expectancy at birth was 37 years. This is a 14-year reduction since 1970. In part this will be due to HIV/AIDS and the social turmoil that has been troubling the country in recent years. The population is 50% syncretic (part Christian part traditional), 25% Christian, 24% indigenous beliefs and 1% Muslim. In the year 2003 the birth rate was 30 per thousand and the death rate 22 per thousand, a rate of natural increase of 0.8%. In 2005 the average woman had 3.4 children and if trends continue the population will be 12.7 million by the year 2050 (Wright 2006: 48).

Contraceptive use increased from 44% of married and cohabiting women in 1990 to over half (54%) in the year 2000 and of these nearly all were modern methods of contraception (UN 2004: 57).

The law on abortion is based on the Termination of Pregnancy Act 1977 which allows abortion on the grounds of the life of the woman, physical or mental defects of the fetus, and rape or incest. Reports suggest that bureaucracy is such that there are many 'black market' abortions (*Global News Update* 2005). UNICEF estimates that there are 70,000 illegal abortions a year and many methods are reported including the consumption of detergents, strong tea, malaria tablets, knitting needles and sharpened reeds. One point made by a leading professor of obstetrics is that people in Zimbabwe (as of 2005) were not aware of the 'morning after' pill which is available in pharmacies (*Global News Update* 2005).

## Conclusion

The evidence shows that Africa has particular problems with family planning as part of wider problems of the health of the continent. The tensions created may be one factor in the cause of wars. There is a great opportunity for the governments on the continent to make important improvements to the lifestyle of its residents and for the richer countries to help in this endeavour.

# LATIN AMERICA
# AND THE CARIBBEAN

*A WOMAN WENT TO HOSPITAL WITH AN
ABORTION AND SHE WAS INFECTED AND
HEMORRHAGING. A DOCTOR STARTED TO
EXAMINE HER AND REALIZED. HE THREW HIS
INSTRUMENTS ON THE FLOOR. HE SAID 'THIS
IS AN ABORTION, YOU GO AHEAD AND DIE.'*

**Human Rights Watch 2007**

Abortion laws throughout most countries in Latin America and the Caribbean are among the most restrictive in the world. With the exception of Barbados, Columbia, Guyana, Puerto Rico and Cuba, which allow legal abortion under a wide range of circumstances, an estimated 95% of abortions in the region are illegal. Even when abortion is legally permitted, safe abortion services are often inaccessible, especially for women who are poor, young or live in rural areas. Though safe abortion services are largely unavailable to most women in the region, an estimated 4.6 million unsafe abortion procedures still occur every year under clandestine conditions, thus highlighting the propensity to have recourse to unsafe abortion when confronted with an unwanted pregnancy.

The unsafe abortion incidence rates are highest in Latin America and the Caribbean. The annual rate of abortion in the region in 2000 was estimated to be 29 unsafe abortions per thousand women aged 15–45. However, the rates of the five countries with estimates range from 12 in the Caribbean to 34 in South America. Similarly, the abortion ratio, which is the number of abortions per hundred pregnancies, is 32 to 100 live births for all of Latin America and the Caribbean, a percentage much higher than in Africa (14 to 100 live births) and comparable with that of South East Asia (23 to 100 live births). The high incidence of unsafe abortion in the region translates into high abortion-related maternal mortality. The unsafe abortion mortality ratio of 30 to 100,000 live births for Latin America and the Caribbean corresponds to about one in six maternal deaths in the region (WHO 2004). Yet another estimate is that in Latin America and the Caribbean unsafe abortion caused 3,700 (17% of) maternal deaths in the year 2000 (WHO 2004: 13).

A study of women's experiences of receiving medical abortion under clinical supervision in Mexico, Colombia, Ecuador and Peru was carried out between October 2003 and May 2004. The fact that such a study could occur suggests that the authorities in these countries were similar to others in the area in turning a 'blind eye' to the issue of abortion. It found that 22 out of the 49 women in the study had never used a modern method of contraception. This indicates that improvement in contraceptive education is very much needed on the continent (Lafaurie et al. 2005). Despite this unmet need population increase has reduced. In the period 1970–1975 the number of children was 5.0 per woman. This fell to 3.7 in the period 1995–2000 (UN 2004: 29). Overall, the main method of contraception on the continent was sterilisation and in 1997 three in ten females were sterilised. One in seven (14%) were using oral contraception. Although the region is predominantly Roman Catholic only one in 20 were using the rhythm method (UN 2004: 47).

The UN subdivides 33 countries of Latin America into three regions. The list is largely of countries with populations above 300,000 and so does not include several smaller countries. The areas are as follows:

- **The Caribbean**   Bahamas, Barbados, Cuba, Dominican Republic, Guadeloupe, Haiti, Jamaica, Martinique, Netherlands Antilles, Puerto Rico, Saint Lucia, Trinidad and Tobago

- **Central America**   Belize, Costa Rica, El Salvador, Guatemala, Honduras, Mexico, Nicaragua, Panama

- **South America**   Argentina, Bolivia, Brazil, Chile, Colombia, Ecuador, French Guiana, Guyana, Paraguay.

There are some difficulties that the region faces and IPPF made the following comments (personal communication):

> While there have been some advances in the provision of adequate reproductive health services in Latin America and the Caribbean since the 1994 International Conference, there are key obstacles which have successfully curtailed expanded access to safe and legal abortion. In particular, a lack of political commitment and policies that are supportive of reproductive health and rights leaves most governments to deny their responsibility to promote safe and legal abortion services. In addition, high levels of social and economic inequalities throughout Latin America and the Caribbean place this region as the highest ranking region for inequalities, placing poverty and the failure of the public sector as tremendous barriers to quality reproductive health care for the most vulnerable and underserved women.

> Further, there has been a rise in very conservative movements in the region whose primary efforts are to block reproductive health services and abortion-related care. Fierce opposition from ultra-conservative religious groups has gained visibility and strength in recent years. The power and the influence of the teachings of the conservative hierarchy of the Catholic Church, in a region that is mostly Catholic, combined with other ultra-conservative religious factions, frame abortion as a mortal sin, and severely damage open public discussion on the issue. This often negatively impacts the willingness of health care providers to provide appropriate care. Additionally, there is ample evidence of the efforts of members of conservative religious organizations such as Opus Dei to occupy key cabinet positions, aggressively working to prevent the passage of legislation that would reform restrictive abortion laws. They wish to establish the right to life at the moment of conception as an integral part of constitutions throughout the region.

Let us consider the different countries in the region concentrating on the larger ones.

## Argentina

The population was estimated at 39.9 million in 2006. Over the period 2000–2005 life expectancy at birth was 74 years. The population is 92% Roman Catholic but fewer than 20% are practising (Wright 2006: 529). Protestants and Jews both comprise 2% of the population which leaves 4% in other religions. In the year 2003 the birth rate was 17 per thousand and the death rate eight per thousand, a rate of natural increase of 0.9%. In 2005 the average woman had 2.3 children and if trends continue the population will be 52.8 million by the year 2050 (Wright 2006: 481). The capital is Buenos Aires which had a population of 13.0 million in the 1991 census.

According to a law passed in the 1880s abortion is illegal in all cases. Exceptions were introduced in 1922 and penalties were suspended in two cases. The law was relaxed where the woman's life or health (including mental health) was threatened and also in the case of rape. The military removed these but when democracy was restored in 1984 they were reinstated except that now abortion for rape was legal only in the case of a mentally incapable woman. Presumably mentally competent women pregnant through rape are obliged to continue the pregnancy. A part of the country's hierarchy is close to the Vatican and in 1998 the president declared that March 25 was to be the 'day of the unborn child'. This is the day when Roman Catholics celebrate the annunciation – when Mary was told she would be the mother of the son of God. There are a number of vibrant women's groups in favour of abortion rights and modern contraception. These include the Catholic Women for the Right to Choose and the Women's Informative Network of Argentina. In 2005 the twentieth annual meeting of women's organisations led to 30,000 marching for the right to choose legal abortion. The health minister, GG Garcia, said he supported legalised abortion, as did Carmen Argibay, who became the first woman appointed to the Argentinean Supreme Court.

The law in Argentina is not observed and in 2004 the health minister estimated that there were 500,000 abortions a year. This is in comparison with a total of 727,000 live births in 2003: according to these figures around two in five pregnancies end in abortion (UN 2007). A 2002 estimate was that 37% of pregnancies end in abortion (Steele and Chiarotti 2004). One woman told how she was offered an abortion for 250 peso but that the cost would be 300 if she wanted antibiotics. A second woman, 36 years old, first became pregnant at the age of 17 and had ten children. She said, 'You seek all the ways out – pills anything. But if there is no way out then you take a knife or a knitting needle.' A third woman went with her friend who had an unwanted pregnancy: 'She went to the illegal clinic and she never came back. They said that it was a problem with the anaesthesia and she died in that very place. They said she died of a heart attack ... legally it was like nothing had happened' (UN 2007). Observers report that women have tried to abort themselves with a variety of things: 'rubber tubes, parsley sticks, knitting needles, and wood'. Many of these abortions are incomplete. Not surprisingly in recent years around 90,000 women are hospitalised annually with the after-effects of unsafe abortion and others neglect to attend through fear of being reported to the police (Berenstein 2006a). A commentator told investigators that many are scared of prison and so die at home. Those who do go to hospital may face unsympathetic treatment. A social worker told Human Rights Watch (2007a): 'A woman went to hospital with an abortion and she was infected and hemorrhaging. A doctor started to examine her and realized. He threw his instruments on the floor. He said "This is an abortion, you go ahead and die." '

Things may have improved after research showed the poor quality of treatment and lack of regard for women, when the ombudsman took action on the issue (Steel and Chiarotti 2004).

Abortion is the major cause of maternal mortality and the rate increased from 38.1 per 100,000 live births in 1997 to 46.1 in 2002 (Human Rights Watch 2007a). In the poorer provinces the rates are much higher and even reach 166 maternal deaths per 100,000 live births (Steel and Chiarotti 2004). There are two approaches to the problem of unsafe abortion. On 18 May 2006 the Christian groups launched a campaign with the slogan 'Adoption not Abortion'. This group seeks to persuade women to continue an unwanted pregnancy instead of seeking a termination, and it wishes the law to remain the same or become more restrictive. Others have been concerned that such a strategy will not work. Berenstein reports that less than two weeks later on 29 May 2006 the campaign for safe abortion launched the second year of its campaign with the slogan: 'Ni una muerto mas por aborto clandestina en Argentina' (No more women dead from clandestine abortions in Argentina). Maria Jose Lubertino, a law professor at Buenos Aires University, said, 'Illegal abortion affects everyone but it kills mainly the poor.' A safe abortion can cost 500 pesos but over six million poor women receive only as much as 65 pesos a month (Berenstein 2006b).

There are signs that the government may at last be recognising the problem. It now provides free contraception for the poor although there are difficulties in access. There is a law review in progress in which abortion is one of a number of issues. In section 93 the proposed code states: 'The woman is not punishable when the abortion occurs with consent of the woman within the first three months of pregnancy as long as the circumstances make it excusable' (Berenstein 2006b). The last phrase restores some ambiguity, but if the law does change unsafe abortion could become a thing of the past.

# Barbados

The population was estimated at 280,000 in 2006. Over the period 2000–2005 life expectancy at birth was 75 years, an increase from 69 in 1970. The population is 67% Protestant, 4% Roman Catholic and 29% none or other (Wright 2006: 487). The capital city is Bridgetown with a population of 6,070 (1990 census) (Wright 2006: 536).

Barbados law was based on that of Britain with the Offences Against the Person Act of 1866 and with the change following the 1938 Bourne case which allowed abortion for rape. In 1983 Barbados liberalised its law similar to the British 1967 Abortion Act to allow a wide range of conditions including taking account of the pregnant woman's social and economic environment. Under the law a pregnancy in the first 12 weeks of pregnancy could have approval for termination by one doctor, for pregnancies of 12–20 weeks two doctors and for those over 20 weeks three doctors. For these later pregnancies abortion would be approved only in the case of risk to the woman's life or 'grave permanent injury to the physical or mental health or the woman or her unborn child'.

IPPF makes the following comments about the country (personal communication):

> Unsafe termination services and its repercussions are common experiences in much of the Caribbean and Latin America. Fortunately, in Barbados safe termination services are widely available since the passing of the 1983 Medical Termination of Pregnancy Act. The existence of the act means Barbados does not have to bear the fallout from high maternal mortality and morbidity rates. The legalization of termination of pregnancy has meant that some of the basic fundamental human rights issues for Barbadian women have been addressed e.g. the right to decide when to have a child and the right to healthcare.

> Within the Barbadian context (as is the experience of many other countries), termination services need to be approached with great sensitivity. Whilst we (as an organisation) are not subject to aggressive confrontation and opposition regarding termination, we are mindful of not attracting unnecessary negative publicity or attracting attention to stigmatise us as 'abortionists'. There is no thriving anti-choice movement in Barbados; although there is a pro-life group in existence which currently demonstrates a limited public presence. Contemporary religious influences, political opinions and attitudes of the media support a pro-choice position. A more heightened awareness of advocating abstinence is emerging and surfacing through many sectors in society but not currently to the exclusion of choice.

> However, a number of barriers exist which inhibit women accessing termination services. The sensitivity of the issue is in itself a barrier as is the existence of traditional attitudes. Furthermore, as termination services are not aggressively marketed in Barbados, many women are not aware of the extent of the comprehensive sexual and reproductive health services that are offered by the Barbados Family Planning Association (BFPA).

> One of the peculiarities of small societies, e.g. Barbados with an approximate population of 270,000, is the feeling that everyone knows or will know your business when you

approach an organisation like the BFPA. There is a very limited pool of people from which employment can be derived, and the likelihood of seeing or meeting your neighbour, friend, family member, church member etc. is high. This again reinforces the feeling that someone other than the people you want to know will know your business. An organisation such as BFPA has to work diligently to develop a trusted reputation for quality confidential care.

There are several options available to women who wish to access abortion services: The BFPA, The Queen Elizabeth Hospital, private gynaecologists, general practitioners, or over the counter purchases from pharmacists. The range of services offered include one or more of the following: surgical or medical termination, pre- and post-termination counselling, infection prevention and integrated family planning and emergency contraception provision.

Presently in Barbados there are no advocacy networks dedicated to the termination of pregnancy. However, the organisations that do exist have their own specific agendas. However, all strongly embrace (a) women's rights to choice, (b) non-discriminatory practices for women, (c) equal access to services, and (d) having primary control over factors that influence their lives. Examples of these include: Caribbean Association for Feminist Research & Action, the Business & Professional Women's Club, Men's Education Support Association, Development Alternative for Women in a New Era (DAWN) and The Bureau of Gender Affairs.

Thus, although Barbados does not give women the express right to choose, its generally liberal attitude means that women have far more legal rights than exist in the majority of countries in the region and consequently it does not have the health problems associated with unsafe abortion.

## Brazil

The population was estimated at 188.1 million in 2006. Over the period 2000–2005 life expectancy at birth was 70 years. The population is 80% Roman Catholic. In the year 2003 the birth rate was 18 per thousand and the death rate six per thousand, a rate of natural increase of 1.2%. In 2005 the average woman had 2.3 children and if trends continue the population will be 233.1 million by the year 2050. The 1991 estimates found the capital, Brasilia, had a population of 1.8 million, smaller than either Sao Paulo at 9.7 million or Rio De Janeiro at 6.0 million (Wright 2006: 543).

The abortion law is based on the 1940 Penal Code and allows abortion to save the life of the woman or for rape, but it is not easy to obtain a legal abortion even for rape. Observers comment: 'Although sexual violence is highly prevalent, legal abortion in cases of rape is rarely performed in public hospitals. This means that a large number of women who should have access to safe abortion in a hospital environment are risking their lives by being forced to resort to clandestine abortions' (Faúndes et al. 2004). During the period 1978–1987 at one Brazilian hospital abortion complications accounted for 47% of maternal deaths (Population Information Program 2007: 1). There was no official sanction of abortion for fetal abnormality so when in July 2004 a judge decided to allow an abortion for anencephaly, a storm broke leading to the Catholic Church strongly challenging the ruling and the case going to the Supreme Court where the judges voted 7–4 to set aside the ruling. Thus, the law is restrictive and in 2004 the country had only 140 legal abortions registered (Ross 2005).

Although legal abortions are few there are many unsafe abortions. It was in August 1986 that Cytotec (misoprostol) was approved for sale over the counter. Word of its abortifacient properties spread until in July 1991 the Brazilian Ministry of Health imposed restrictions (Arilha and Barbosa 1993). This meant that many women seeking abortions had to return to traditional methods. Also in 1991 the Guttmacher Institute estimated that the country had 1.4 million (with a range of from 1.0 million to 2.0 million) abortions, an abortion rate of 41 per thousand women aged 15–44 and one-quarter of pregnancies ending in abortion (Henshaw et al. 1999). Later observers put the number of abortions as between 1 and 1.4 million (Goldman et al. 2005; Ross 2005). The Health Ministry reported that in 2001 there were 242,000 cases of women attending hospital following an illegal abortion. This was a reduction from the 1991 figure of 289,000 (Henshaw et al. 1999). Dulce Xavier of Brazil's chapter of Catholics for a Free Choice commented:

> Here in Brazil, women sometimes ingest a poison used to kill rats... It's a dramatic situation and the women who die as a result of clandestine abortions in Brazil are mainly young, black and poor. Women with money can pay to have an abortion in a private clinic (Ross 2005).

In a study, over 4,000 Brazilian gynaecologists were asked about their personal experience of abortion: almost a quarter of female gynaecologists and a third of male gynaecologists had encountered an unwanted pregnancy and four out of five of these were aborted (Faúndes et al. 2004: 47). Even amongst those to whom religion was 'very important', still 70% of unwanted pregnancies were aborted. Observers have reported the individual problems women have faced. Ross reports a woman identified only as Martha, a 26-year-old mother, who had been raped by her estranged husband. Marital rape was not recognised in Brazilian law and her husband threatened to report her to the police. Nevertheless, she could not face continuing the pregnancy under these circumstances. She used Cytotec, which precipitated the abortion but left her bleeding for 40 days. She did not go to the hospital for fear of being prosecuted. Another woman had greater problems. In the autumn of 2002, Viviane Coutino, a breastfeeding mother, became pregnant again and took Cytotec. She became ill and checked into hospital where the following occurred:

> An attending physician angry about the steady stream of abortion he was seeing accused her of infanticide a crime carrying a possible six year prison term. Police handcuffed Coutino still bleeding from the abortion to the hospital bed. Later in the day they booked her into Rio de Janeiro's notorious Bangu prison. She spent nearly two months in jail. She never knew who was caring for her 10 month old son. She said 'I could not believe this was happening. I thought only about my son' (Hall 2003).

Although, poor women may fall foul of the law, it seems that in Brazil there is a network of doctors providing abortions for richer women. When considering the role of abortifacient drugs, observers noted that there were separate gynaecologists for general needs and for abortions. In part this was because doctors performing abortions have to 'pay police in order to obtain a corrupt form of authorisation' (Arilha and Barbosa 1993: 45). When Cytotec was approved many regular gynaecologists began to become involved with abortion.

There has been some liberalisation in observance of the law. At one time the woman had to file a complaint to the police in order to obtain an abortion for rape. This requirement has now been removed. Furthermore, the leftist government of da Silva in April 2005 set up a tripartite commission to consider changes to the law (Ross 2005).

## Caribbean Islands of Anguilla, Antigua, St Kitts, St Martin and Sint Maarten

These five countries are relatively small with a total population of about 200,000 and they are situated in the north-east Caribbean. St Martin and Sint Maarten (French) is a two-country island where Pheterson and Azize began researching and as the project developed, the other countries were added. Anguilla is a British Overseas Territory; Antigua is part of the two-island country of Antigua and Barbuda which has been independent since 1981. St Kitts is one of the two islands in St Kitts and Nevis, independent since 1983 (Pheterson and Azize 2005). Research was in large part based on the information from 16 abortion providers, only two of which were complying with legal guidelines, and a further 30 health professionals, advisors or government officials including a minister of health and an attorney general (Pheterson and Azize 2005: 45).

At Sint Martin the researchers went to the Woman's Desk, a government community centre, and were told:

> Abortion is illegal in Sint Maarten ... no the law is not a problem ... Everyone knows who is doing them. We don't talk about it, we can't talk about it since it is illegal and we are a Government agency. Abortion is a taboo here. (Pheterson and Azize 2005: 46)

A physician told them that abortion was tolerated because people knew it was legal in Holland. Another respondent, who provided aspiration abortions, told how when an inspector from the Ministry of Health inspected all they did was asked about his technique. He commented: 'They know it is a needed service.' A fourth doctor said that he was not in favour of legalisation because it would lead to greater bureaucracy and delays. 'The system works fine the way it is.'

In the French part of the island the service depended on French law and was the only one of the five countries to provide medical abortion with the combination of mifepristone and misoprostol. At the time of the study this had to be carried out in a hospital rather than at home or in a doctor's office. In 2004 French practice changed to allow doctors to supervise medical abortions up to 49 days from last menstrual period. The researchers reported that some migrant women were buying misoprostol from underground distributors who carried the drug from one island to another. Some local residents told that women from Anguilla would go to St Martin to avoid trouble from their church which might expel them if it were discovered. Anguilla had changed its law soon before the research began but it does not seem that this liberalisation had much effect on practice at the time.

In Antigua abortion remained illegal, although it was carried out openly. A nurse who had learned to do manual vacuum aspiration said that once abortions were carried out by unskilled operators:

> People used to end up with sepsis really sick and when I say sick I have seen times you had to stay outside the room the smell was so bad. You don't see that anymore. Doctors realised that people were dying or becoming infertile and they decided was inhumane to let people suffer like that ... now people go to the doctors and the doctors help them. The

> Church doesn't say anything about it because it isn't legal … but it's done as a cloak and
> dagger thing, its done more or less openly and safely (Pheterson and Azize 2005).

One gynaecologist told how when doctors approached the government to attempt to change the law it responded: 'Look, it hasn't been a problem, what we do is turn a blind eye, but to legislate that abortion would be legal would cause too much a problem with the Church.' Another respondent, who was a health administrator for a non-government organisation, said he thought the country was not ready for reform and expressed the view that stirring up a debate would damage the provision of services (Pheterson and Azize 2005: 48).

Another gynaecologist told how he had worked in many of the English speaking Caribbean islands and abortion was not legal in most of them with Barbados and Guyana being exceptions. However, he commented, 'It's tolerated because nobody is going to prosecute a doctor' (Pheterson and Azize 2005 48). In May 2005 the researchers organised a conference in Antigua-Barbuda: 'Safe Abortion in the Caribbean: From Law to Practice'. Participants attended from 14 Caribbean countries including Barbados, Curaçao, Dominica, Guadeloupe, Guyana, Jamaica, St Eustatius, Puerto Rico, and St Kitts-Nevis, St Lucia and Trinidad-Tobago. The conference recommended decriminalisation of abortion in the Caribbean.

## Chile

The population was estimated at 16.1 million in 2006. Over the period 2000–2005 life expectancy at birth was 78 years. The population is 90% Roman Catholic. In the year 2003 the birth rate was 16 per thousand and the death rate six per thousand, a rate of natural increase of 1.0%. In 2005 the average woman had 2.0 children and if trends continue the population will be 21.8 million by the year 2050. The capital, Gran Santiago, has a population of 5.1 million (1995 estimate).

Chile is one of three countries which do not officially allow abortion to save the life of the woman. It is based on the 1874 Penal Code which did not allow abortion for any reason. In 1931 there was liberalisation and abortion was allowed to save the life of the woman, but in 1989 General Pinochet's regime repealed even this minor liberalisation. During the presidential elections of 1999 President Lagos supported abortion to save the life of the woman and for her health, but he later retracted from this position (Human Rights Watch 2007b). We saw in the Introduction that for the first half of the nineteenth century the Catholic Church did not allow abortion for an ectopic pregnancy. Although it changed its view, the Chilean government has not acted on it. Observers state that the law will not allow an immediate abortion but requires waiting until the final stages of pregnancy before termination (Human Rights Watch 2007a).

In 1964 there were 118 deaths recorded per 100,000 live births by unsafe abortion. The government then began to promote contraception. The maternal death rate from illegal operations fell to under a quarter of its previous level to 24 deaths in 1979. This reduction in deaths may also have been due to improvements in the care of abortion complications. More recent data shows that the maternal mortality has declined from 22.3 per 100,000 women aged 15–44 in 1997 to 16.7 in 2002 (Human Rights Watch 2007A).

In 1990 Chile was held to have an estimated 160,000 abortions each year, a rate of 50 per thousand women aged 15–44 and over three times the world average abortion rate (Henshaw et al. 1999). This figure seems to have been widely accepted and some later authorities are still quoting the figure of 160,000 (e.g. Estrada 2006), although the government quotes a figure of 130,000 unsafe abortions a year and 32,000 women hospitalised by complications (White 2006).

There have been reductions in the maternal mortality rates. In the period 1990–2000 the overall maternal mortality rate fell by 60.3% and a large but unspecified part of this fall will have been due to a reduction in deaths from unsafe abortion. The maternal mortality rate from illegal abortion fell from 22.3 in 1997 to 16.7 per 100,000 births. Although deaths from unsafe abortion have reduced they are still much higher than elsewhere and women are facing great difficulties. Ross reports the case of 16-year-old Monica Maureira, admitted to hospital haemorrhaging, who said, 'I remember the nurses telling me that if I did not give them the name of the doctor who gave me the abortion, then they would let me bleed to death' (Ross 2006).

It appears that there is still a large problem with teenage pregnancy; Ross, writing in 2006, reported that 14% of children were mothers by the age of 14. This led on 30 Jan 2006 to the president, Michelle Bachelet, legalising the 'morning after' pill for teenagers without parental consent, but this law was set aside later in the year at the Santiago Court of Appeals when opponents argued that there should be parental consent for the ages 14–18 years (Ross 2006). The court then changed its mind and these pills are again allowed without parental consent. This could help reduce the number of unsafe abortions.

An important ten-year project led by Ramiro Molina of the University of Chile introduced contraception, counselling and education to three poor communities. This led to an 82% drop in the abortion rate in some communities. This project has been used as an example of what could be done to improve women's health (Ross 2005). Although Chile is strongly Catholic, a study found that over four out of five (81.3%) Catholics were in favour of artificial contraception (CIA 2007), so a movement for modern contraceptive coverage may find support. There is less possibility of abortion liberalisation. Estrada in 2006 wrote an article entitled: 'Chile: therapeutic abortion a distant but not impossible prospect'. She pointed out that activists fighting for liberalisation faced a difficult situation with zero political support, the opposition of the Catholic Church and limited public support. However, she noted the importance of the 1979 UN General Assembly 'Convention on the elimination of all forms of discrimination against women' (CEDAW). Chile ratified this in 1989 but has not ratified the optional protocol which recognises the competence of CEDAW to receive and study individual complaints. This, she says, had been 'bogged down' in Congress since 2002 (Estrada 2006).

## Colombia

The population was estimated at 43.6 million in 2006. Over the period 2000–2005 life expectancy at birth was 72 years. The population is 90% Roman Catholic. In the year 2003 the birth rate was 22 per thousand and the death rate six per thousand, a rate of natural increase of 1.6%. In 2005 the average woman had 2.5 children and if trends continue the population will be 21.8 million by the year 2050. In 1998 the maternal mortality rate was 71 but it had risen to 99 by 2001 (Human Rights Watch 2007c). The capital, Bogota, has a population of 5.2 million (1995 estimate) (Wright 2006: 557). Contraceptive use increased from two-thirds (66%) of married and cohabiting women in 1990 to 77% in the year 2000 and of these 64% were modern methods of contraception (UN 2004: 57).

The law of abortion in Colombia dates back at least to 1936 although the penalty was lower for women who had abortions 'to protect their honor' (Human Rights Watch 2007c). In 1979 the congresswoman, Consuela Lleras, unsuccessfully submitted a bill to legalise abortions on three grounds. These were for maternal health, rape or incest, or fetal abnormality (Vieira 2005). Since then there have been several other bills, but until 2006 Colombia was recognised as one of the three countries in Latin America not to allow any abortions – the others being Chile and El Salvador. This led to high numbers of illegal abortion and between 1985 and 1989 unsafe abortion accounted for nearly one-third of maternal deaths at one Columbian hospital (Population Information Program 2007).

In 1994 the Constitutional Court ruled that the general prohibition on abortion was constitutional. Despite the general illegality of abortion often being mentioned in the literature of those on both sides of the debate, the overall prohibition had been softened in 1991 when four Constitutional Court judges commented about women pregnant through rape: 'The exceptional and admirable thing would be for the woman to decide to continue the pregnancy until she gave birth … But she cannot be required to procreate, nor can she be the object of penal sanctions for having exercised her fundamental rights.'

In 2005 a lawyer, Monica Roa, with the support of the Spanish- based group Woman's Link Worldwide challenged the law. On 10 May 2006 the Constitutional Court voted by five to three that abortion was not a crime under the three conditions maternal health, rape or incest, or fetal abnormality that Llera had tried to have inserted in the law 27 years earlier. The conditions meant that it might still be difficult to obtain a legal abortion. To obtain an abortion for rape the woman had to file a police report, and to obtain one on the grounds of health she needed a medical certificate. The ruling explicitly stated that international laws take precedence over national ones. The Catholic Church excommunicated the five judges who voted for the change in the law (Gumbel 2006). One case that was given great publicity while the Court was considering its decision was that of Marta Gonzalez, a 34-year-old mother of four children. Three weeks into her pregnancy she was diagnosed with cancer and wished to have an abortion so that she could have chemotherapy and radiation. This was refused by the authorities and as her pregnancy was logged in the system no private hospital would go against the decision. She had to endure lack of treatment (Gumbel 2006).

The first abortion carried out under the act gained great publicity. An 11-year-old girl was pregnant after being raped by her stepfather. There were hundreds of opponents to the act outside the hospital and the Catholic Church announced it was to excommunicate all those involved in the girl's abortion including judges, physicians, nurses and the girl's parents.

In 1989 it was estimated that there were 289,000 abortions (with a range 288,000–404,000), an abortion rate of 36.3 per thousand women of fertile age. In that year 58,000 women were recorded as being hospitalised owing to incomplete abortion (Henshaw et al. 1999). More recently there are an estimated 300,000 illegal abortions each year. It is calculated that 36% of teenager pregnancies end in abortion compared with 12% of pregnancies in married women (Human Rights Watch 2007c).

# Cuba

The population was estimated to be 11.3 million in 2006 and it is the most populous country in the Caribbean. Over the period 2000–2005 life expectancy at birth was 77 years. The population was at least 85% Roman Catholic before Castro came to power and promoted a variant of Marxism which led to atheism being promoted. There is a strong Protestant minority with 300,000 members in 54 different denominations. In 1999 the Pope visited Cuba and publicly confronted Castro on the issue of religious freedom (Wright 2006: 563). In the year 2003 the birth rate was 12 per thousand and the death rate seven per thousand, a rate of natural increase of 0.5%. In 2005 the average woman had 1.6 children and if trends continue the population will reduce to 10.1 million by the year 2050. The capital, Havana, has a population of 2.2 million. Although the country pays lip service to Marxism, like the Soviet Union before, it does not follow his belief in the 'withering away of the state'; rather it has kept strong central control. An example of this is that Cuba compulsorily tested all its citizens for HIV and those who tested positive were taken to Los Cocos and not allowed to leave. This policy was discontinued in the 1990s, but in 2003 Cuba had the lowest HIV prevalence in the Americas – 0.1% – which is less than one-tenth of the next lowest country in the Caribbean. The country has the second highest ratio of doctors in the world with only Italy having a higher proportion.

From 1870 until 1936 the abortion laws were those inherited from Spain, but in 1936 there was liberalisation and abortion was allowed on a range of grounds including to save the life or health of the woman, rape, and abduction not followed by marriage. Abortions became available in private clinics (Babablu 2004). Abortion has been legal on request up to the tenth week of pregnancy since 1965. After that it is allowed for medical reasons (Acosta 2007). The abortion rate is high and some local observers comment that many young people prefer abortion to oral contraception, IUD or condoms. A 21-year-old student who had had two abortions commented: 'Something always gave, you either forgot one of the pills or the condoms broke.' In 1996, 209,900 abortions were reported with a rate of 77.7 per thousand women aged 15–44 (Henshaw et al. 1999).

The relatively high abortion rate can be attributed in part to the scarcity of contraceptives which, like other important products, are often unavailable.

## Mexico

The population was estimated at 107.5 million in 2006. Over the period 2000–2005 life expectancy at birth was 75 years. The population is 89% Roman Catholic and 6% Protestant. In the year 2003 the birth rate was 22 per thousand and the death rate five per thousand, a rate of natural increase of 1.7%. In 2005 the average woman had 2.2 children and if trends continue the population will be 140.2 million by the year 2050. Family size used to be much larger and in the 1970s the average woman had 6.8 children (del Carmen Elu 1993). Mexico has a federal policy and consists of 31 states and the Federal District. The capital is Mexico City which in the 1990 census had a population of 8.2 million (Wright 2006: 486). Contraceptive use increased from below three in five (58%) married and cohabiting women in 1990 to 75% in the year 2000 and of these 66% were using modern methods of contraception (UN 2004: 57).

Mexico criminalised abortion in 1931. There are exceptions for the life of the woman, rape and the curious case 'where the abortion is the result of negligent behaviour of the pregnant woman'. Another curiosity of the Mexican law is that there is a lower penalty for abortion with a maximum sentence of one year for a woman 'who does not have a bad reputation' (Human Rights Watch 2007d). A major change occurred in April 2007 when Mexico City decided to make abortion legal on request in the first trimester. This will clearly have a great effect in the future.

There is evidence of a growth in contraception use and while 30% of married women were using it in 1976, it increased to 48% in 1982 and 53% in 1987. Female sterilisation grew from 9% in 1976 to 36% of married women in 1987 (del Carmen Elu 1993).

Illegal abortion has been common for some time. In 1989 the police stormed an abortion clinic and detained eight women with a resultant series of protests (del Carmen Elu 1993). In 1990 it was estimated there were 533,000 abortions annually (with a range 297,000–746,000) giving a rate of 25.1 per thousand women of fertile age (Henshaw et al. 1999). In 1991 in Mexico City observers report one in two of the women hospitalised were there through induced abortion (del Carmen Elu 1993). In 2003 the Autonomous New University of Mexico estimated that there were half a million legal and illegal abortions a year. In 2005 it admitted it had underestimated and revised its figure and estimated that there were approaching a million abortions a year which would be around 30% of pregnancies. The government had estimated a lower figure of 100,000 unsafe operations in 1995. It deems that abortion has been increasing because the maternal mortality rate of the country rose from 37 per 100,000 live births to 64 between 1997 and 2002 (Human Rights Watch 2007d). The fact that abortion is cheaper in Mexico has meant that some US women travelled there for abortion after financial support was denied to US women during the presidency of Jimmy Carter. Feminists in the USA were angry about the decision and especially so when a woman died in Mexico. (Her death inspired a book entitled *Rosie, the Investigation of a Wrongful Death*.) There is also evidence of richer Mexican women travelling to the USA for abortions.

Although abortion is legal for rape it has often proved difficult for women to obtain. A major report on the issue told of one 13-year-old girl pregnant by a family member who was made to watch a factually inaccurate film by a social worker. Others had had abortion refused. In one such case a 16-year-old was raped weekly by her father. She said in her evidence (Human Rights Watch 2007d):

> Then my father took me to a hostel. He penetrated me and it hurt a lot when he penetrated me. I cried and I said to my father that it hurt a lot. I want to declare that I don't want to have the child I am expecting, because I won't be able to love it because it is my father's.

This led to Kenneth Roth of Human Rights Watch commenting: 'Pregnant rape victims are essentially assaulted twice – first by the perpetrators who rape them and then by the public figures that ignore them, insult them and deny them a legal abortion.' It could be that a court case could lead to changes. A 13-year-old girl by the name of Paulina had been raped in her own home by a heroin addict and denied an abortion. In 2002 the Mexico government was taken to the Inter American Commission for Human Rights and in March 2006 the Mexican government agreed to pay Paulina reparation and legal costs of $40,000 and to pay for the education of her son. In addition they issued a decree to its abortion providers giving new guidelines as to how to treat rape victims. One hopes that the situation as regards rape will improve (Illingworth 2006).

The Secretariat of Health in Mexico has reported 300,000 legal abortions a year, which seems high given the difficulties in obtaining an abortion even for rape (Illingworth 2006). The system in Mexico could mean that women are travelling to more liberal states for abortion as happened in the USA with the NY State decision in 1970.

There is some evidence of improved use of contraception, which is likely to have reduced the number of abortions. There is an organisation openly in favour of women's right to choose and other pressure groups in addition to the Mexican chapter of Catholics for a Free Choice. These could have a greater effect in future years (Illingworth 2006). An opinion poll in the year 2000 showed that 76% of 3,000 respondents aged 15–65 agreed with abortion for the woman's health. It also showed that most Mexican Catholics believed the Church's and legislators' personal religious beliefs should not be a factor in abortion legislation (Garcia et al. 2004).

## Peru

The population was estimated at 28.3 million in 2006 and it claims to be the nineteenth largest country in the world. Over the period 2000–2005 life expectancy at birth was 70 years. The population is 90% Roman Catholic. In the year 2003 the birth rate was 23 per thousand and the death rate six per thousand, a rate of natural increase of 1.6%. In 2005 the average woman had 2.8 children and if trends continue the population will be 41.1 million by the year 2050. There are high rates of teenage pregnancy: 32% of women give birth while still in their teens (International Women's Health Coalition 2007). The capital city, Lima, has a population of 5.7 million (Wright 2006: 650). Contraceptive use increased from over half (54%) of married and cohabiting women in 1990 to seven out of ten (69%) in the year 2000 and of these 50% were using modern methods of contraception (UN 2004: 57).

The abortion law in Peru allows the operation to save the woman's life and in order to protect the woman's physical and mental health. Some of the interpretations of the law have come under criticism. In one case KL, a 17-year-old, underwent a scan and anencephaly was diagnosed. Despite the fact that this condition is fatal to the child, she was denied an abortion and was forced to care for the baby for the four days until it died. The case resulting from this event led to its being the first case for the United Nations Human Rights Committee. It ruled that the government 'in denying access to legal abortion violates a woman's basic human rights'. This was the first time that an international human rights body had held a government responsible for failing to secure access to a legal abortion. The *New York Times* carried the story (17 November 2005) under the headline 'Woman forced to carry fatally impaired fetus to term wins case'. Luisa Cabal commented on the case:

> Every woman who lives in any of the 154 countries that are part of this treaty – including the US – now has a legal tool to use in defense of her rights. When abortion is legal it is the government's duty to ensure that women have access to it.

On the 22 October 2003 Susan Chavez gave a briefing to the US Congress about the effects of the gag rule. She said it led to an increase in unsafe abortions and reported:

> A woman was recently found buried in an abandoned lot on the outskirts of Lima. She had been dead for several months and had died from the complications of an unsafe abortion. No one ever claimed the woman's body and she remained unaccounted for in the statistics.

She carried on to state that in Peru there are 85,000 women who are sexually active, of reproductive age, who do not want children and yet have no access to contraception. This is a quarter of all women in this group. There is thus a need for more resources. She commented further that the gag rule was denying funds and causing preventable deaths by blocking non-governmental organisations from improving access to safe abortion in cases where it is legal. The gag rule prevents people even talking about abortion which led to Chavez commenting: 'You in the US have very active debates on abortion and your women are not dying from unsafe abortion. For us it seems very hypocritical. Three women a day die needlessly' (Chavez 2003).

In 1989 it was estimated there were 271,150 unsafe abortions a year giving a rate of 56.1 per thousand women of fertile age. In this year 55,000 women were hospitalised (Henshaw et al. 1999). The average number of abortions per year was stated as being 1.8 per woman. A later estimate is that in more recent, but unspecified, years there were 410,000 unsafe abortions every year (International Women's Health Coalition 2007). This led to the country having the third highest rate of maternal mortality in Latin America and the Caribbean: nearly one-third of the pregnancy-related maternal deaths were due to unsafe abortion. Chavez (2003) commented on the situation: 'Clandestine abortion continues to be one of the main ways women control their health.'

One of the organisations working in Peru is Pathfinder International. As seen in the Introduction the organisation challenged the gag rule, and although it lost the case it nevertheless won some useful concessions. These enabled it to improve aftercare in the case of unsafe abortions and to provide contraceptive advice after birth or abortion (Webb 2000). One part of its programme was to promote manual vacuum aspiration (MVA); it completed a module on this in 1999. It arranged training for doctors and nurses and found MVA was more effective than dilatation and curettage (D&C) for after-abortion care. In Peru in 1995 the cost of a D&C was $68 while that of MVA was only $16. Nurses commented that the training had created an atmosphere in which they were no longer afraid to display empathy towards the patient. Pathfinder worked with the government of Peru and by 1993 had trained 3,800 doctors and nurses in post-abortion aftercare for MVA (Webb 2000). In 1997 the British government also financed educational programmes. In 2007 Milka Dinev and colleagues reported that in 2005–2006, 1,565 women attending for abortion were offered either two 800 ml doses of misoprostol separated by 24 hours or MVA (personal communication). A total of 812 chose the medical abortion option and 753 MVA. The medical option was 80% successful and when it did not work MVA was provided. Dinev and colleagues commented: 'High quality service can be provided in countries with restrictive laws.'

There has been other activity for change in Peru. The organisation Flora Tristan, a Peruvian feminist organisation, was founded in 1979 and recently has been co-ordinating an international campaign to legalise abortion around the world. The September 28 (1990) campaign in particular aims to decriminalise abortion in Latin America and the Caribbean.

## Puerto Rico

The population was estimated at 3.9 million in 2006. The population is 85% Roman Catholic and 15% Protestant and other. In the year 2003 the birth rate was 14 per thousand and the death rate eight per thousand, a rate of natural increase of 0.6%. In 2005 the average woman had 1.9 children and if trends continue the population will be 4.8 million by the year 2050 (Wright 2006: 483). The capital city is San Juan with a population of 422,000 (2000 census). Puerto Rico is an autonomous political entity in voluntary association with the USA. Its constitution came in to effect on 22 July 1952 when it changed from being a US colony. Its political structure is modelled on that of the USA and it too celebrates US Independence Day (4 July). Contraceptive services in the country date back to 1925 when Dr José Rolon had contacts with the US activist

Margaret Sanger, who in turn had close links with the British proponents. One of the aims was to reduce the incidence of illegal abortion. The first clinic was opened in the city of Ponce and several more followed until in the 1930s they were briefly closed after pressure from the Catholic Church which opposed both contraception and abortion. In the 1950s oral contraception was first tested in Puerto Rico before it was legalised in the United States and Britain. Historically, there have been strong sex distinctions with men being expected to express machismo and women to play the subservient role. Maria is by far the most common name and in some families more than one daughter might even be so named with an alternative as a second name. This is presumably to remind women of the Virgin Mary and her acceptance of her lot. A perhaps surprising finding by numerous researchers is that Catholics use contraception and abortion just as much as non-Catholics. In 1990 there were an estimated 50,000 to 75,000 abortions every year though it is not clear why there is not a more accurate figure when abortion is legal (Montesinos and Preciado 2007).

IPPF commentators state (personal communication):

> Over 30% of families receive some kind of social assistance from the government. More than 450,000 families are living below the poverty-line and 60% of homes where women are the heads of household live below the poverty-line. According to the vital statistics issued by the Department of Health in 2002, 52,871 babies were born that year. The infant mortality rate was 9.8 per thousand. Overall 1.4% of babies were born with low birth weights and infant mortality resulting from low birth weight accounted for 70% of infant deaths.

> A study by the Department of Health in 2003 showed that 39% of women plan their pregnancies. In younger age groups, the percentage was much lower. Another study by the University of Puerto Rico found that 78% of women with partners use contraceptive methods and almost 45% of women were sterilized. In terms of youth under the age of 19, 36% were sexually active; this age group accounted for almost 20% of all births. Abortion has been legal in Puerto Rico since the Supreme Court of the United States ruled on the Roe v. Wade case (1973). In the cases of Montalvo v. Colón (1974) and Pueblo v. Duarte Mendoza (1980), the Supreme Court of Puerto Rico reiterated the applicability of Roe v. Wade (1973). This case determined that women's right to abortion was based on the constitutional right to privacy. The Pueblo v. Duarte case not only reinforced the legality of abortion in Puerto Rico, but also ruled that there are no legal restrictions or limits on when it can be practiced during the gestation period. Since then, in Puerto Rico the number of cases of clinical complications resulting from unsafe abortions has decreased. In 2001, approximately 13,800 abortions were recorded in seven clinics in Puerto Rico, and it is estimated that over 2,000 abortions were performed by physicians in private practice. The abortion rate is lower in Puerto Rico than in the US and other countries in Latin America and the Caribbean. There are three main reasons for this fact. First more than 45% of women in reproductive age are sterilized, secondly, oral contraceptives are widely used and thirdly abortion services are costly.

> The Second National Survey on Abortion in Puerto Rico, conducted by Prof. Yamila Azize, shows the lack of knowledge among various groups on the legality of abortion. These include one-third of women who have had an abortion, 50% of staff at family planning clinics and 45% of university students. This same survey showed that 86% of gynecology and obstetrics students did not know minors' rights or the trimester system.

The mere fact that abortion is legal in Puerto Rico is not enough if the government, NGOs, doctors, universities and other health-based organizations are not involved in the process of educating and informing the general public about abortion, especially women. Some of the barriers to accessing safe abortion services in Puerto Rico include: lack of information on its legal status, lack of skilled and available providers, the high cost of the services, the few private alternatives available, the fact that the government will only provide services in cases of rape or if a woman's life is at risk, stigmatization, moral or religious values, and the fact that only nine clinics are certified. Particularly for young women, the primary limitation is that most service providers require the presence of an adult. For young women, cost is also one of the major barriers to access. Moreover, seven of the nine public clinics that currently offer abortion services are in the metropolitan area, limiting access to women in rural areas or in other areas of the country. The other two clinics are in the southern and northwestern parts of the country.

# Uruguay

The population was estimated at 3.4 million in 2006. Over the period 2000–2005 life expectancy at birth was 75 years. The population is 66% Roman Catholic, 2% Protestant and 1% Jewish, although fewer than half the population attend worship regularly. In the year 2003 the birth rate was 17 per thousand and the death rate nine per thousand, a rate of natural increase of 0.8%. In 2005 the average woman had 2.2 children and if trends continue the population will be 4.1 million by the year 2050 (Wright 2006: 489). In the 1970s the country was under a military regime and was reported to have the highest number of political prisoners in proportion to the population. In 1980 Uruguayans rejected army rule and a slow process began leading to civilian presidential elections in 1984 (Wright 2006: 700). Abortion has been illegal since 1938 in Uruguay and a commentator said about the decision: 'The abortion law was not the result of serious debate but of trivial discussion while approving the national budget for the year' (Choike 2002). An unusual feature of the law is that 'no economic or social justification makes an abortion legal but when such a defense is offered, the penalty for breaking the law is waived'. There is also the provision that an abortion can be allowed in the case of 'the jeopardy of a man's honor' (Choike 2002). Since military rule ended there have been numerous attempts to liberalise the law and since 1998 there has been a big movement to change the law. One such attempt to change the law in 2002 saw a bill approved by the House of Representatives in December by 47 votes to 40 with ten representatives not voting, but the Senate blocked the legislation. It faced great opposition from the Catholic Church which read out the names of those voting for the act at mass. Furthermore five Republican senators from the USA led by Chris Smith sent faxes to the senators urging them to oppose the act. The Methodists were more supportive and on 11 February 2003 the Evangelical Methodist Church of Uruguay published a statement on abortion:

> The Methodist church does not condone abortion or anything else that attacks human life. However, we must not fall into the trap of confusing decriminalization with inciting or promoting abortion (Methodist Church 2003).

It continued to say that there would be two positive factors to emerge from a liberalisation of the law. The first is that it would clearly improve the overall health of women who would not have to undergo illegal operations and secondly it would help to reduce discrimination against women (Methodist Church 2003).

In the end it failed. However, in 2004 a relaxation occurred when the Ministry of Public Health approved a measure which allows doctors to give advice to women who want abortions. It hoped that this change would result in a reduction in problems from unsafe abortions. There is a movement to liberalise the law and Senator Margarita Percovich said in January that she and her colleagues were planning a new bill for 2007 which she hoped would succeed because 'this time abortion is to be put as a matter of human rights rather than one of health care' (Catholic News Agency 2007). Sara Bossio, who took the post of Chief Justice of Uruguay's Supreme Court, made it clear that she wanted change. In particular she said she was worried about poor women: 'They have many kids and they have no way to obtain abortions, while women who are well off can go to any clinic and get one' (CAN/LW News 2007). Reports stated that there would be an attempt to bring in abortion on request later in 2007.

An estimate relating to 2002 suggested that each year there were 30,000–50,000 abortions. Until legalisation, unsafe abortions will continue. In 2004 the *New Internationalist* reported that abortion caused 47% of the maternal deaths at the leading maternity hospital (Pereira Rossell) compared with 28% in the rest of the country, 24% in Latin America and 13% worldwide. It also gave details of a case which shows the problems with the law not clearly giving women the right to choose an abortion:

> Flavia was 16 and had a six month old baby that she was still breastfeeding at night. She had no access to sex education or abortion clinics; and only an abortion pill that she put in her vagina. Rosario Echargue was the doctor who received her at the hospital an hour after she had used the pill. 'She had a pain in her stomach abundant diarrhea and unstoppable vomiting. She was pale and trembling, did not understand what was happening to her. She died and she was not even pregnant' (Fonseca and Pujol 2004).

IPPF states that there is no data on morbidity in the country, although there is an estimate that for each death due to unsafe abortion, there are ten women with complications and 100 with minimal consequences. Senator A Couriel stated that for every death there are many women whose condition is so dire that they will never have a child.

Whether a new bill passes remains to be seen but two commentators stated: 'When a country advances in recognition of sexual and reproductive rights the whole country advances. As women advance democracy is strengthened and citizenship is built' (Fonseca and Pujol 2004).

## Venezuela

The population was estimated at 25.7 million in 2006. Over the period 2000–2005 life expectancy at birth was 73 years. The population is nominally 96% Roman Catholic and 2% Protestant. In the year 2003 the birth rate was 20 per thousand and the death rate five per thousand, a rate of natural increase of 1.5%. In 2005 the average woman had 2.6 children and if trends continue the population will be 41.7 million by the year 2050 (Wright 2006: 483). The evidence shows that since 1970 the average family size has declined from 5.9 children per woman, so a future reduction in birth rate is likely. The capital city is Caracas with a population of 3.4 million.

Under the Criminal Code of 1964 abortion was illegal in Venezuela except to save the life of the woman. Legal abortion needs the written consent of the woman, her husband or a legal representative. In 1986 there was a proposal for reform to permit abortion for therapeutic grounds such as the woman's physical or mental health or rape, incest and eugenics. This law has not yet been incorporated. In 2005 supporters of President Hugo Chavez unsuccessfully lobbied for abortion on the grounds of rape and incest (Population Division 2007h).

Illegal abortion accounted for 24.6% of the maternal deaths in Venezuela in 1980–1983 but this had reduced to 13.6% in 1995. This seems largely to be due to the reduction in demand for abortion because of improved birth control but it may also reflect improved treatment. The government believes that the abortion problem 'can be alleviated by the increased provisions of family life education and family planning services'. The government has also created the Ministry of the Family which is the first institution of its kind in Latin America.

The president of Venezuela, Hugo Chavez, is a maverick who is friendly with the Cubans and very critical of the USA's interventionist policies; there is much discussion of the possibility of a US invasion of the country. A bizarre incident occurred when the US right-wing evangelist Pat Robertson called for the assassination of Chavez who in return called for Robertson's extradition.

## Conclusion

The evidence of Latin America shows strongly the effect of the Catholic Church with many countries showing evidence of lack of modern contraception and abortion that is illegal. The evidence from the continent shows that there is a relationship in that those countries with legal abortion have fewer unsafe abortions and health problems for women in comparison with those where abortion is only allowed on restricted grounds.

The recent change in the law in Mexico City could have important and long-lasting effects. The advent of medical abortion and greater access to medical vacuum aspiration could have an important influence on future developments.

# OCEANIA

*MANY PEOPLE BELIEVE PREGNANCY
WILL NOT OCCUR UNTIL COUPLES HAVE
SEX AT LEAST SIX TIMES.*

**Olivier Miller personal
communication 2004**

The continent had an estimated 30,000 unsafe abortions in the year 2,000 which gave it an abortion rate of 17 per thousand women aged 15–44 years. Oceania's population growth has reduced in recent years. In the period 1970–1975 it was 5.8 children per woman and fell to 2.5 in the period 1990–1995 and to 2.4 from 1995 to 2000 (UN 2004: 29). In the two richer countries in the region – Australia and New Zealand – the birth rate declined from 2.6 per woman in 1970–1975 to 1.8 in 1995–2000. In Melanesia the number of children per woman is more than double this and in 1995–2000 there were 4.4 births per woman (UN 2004: 29).

The countries are:

- **Australia**, New Zealand
- **Melanesia, Micronesia, Polynesia**   Fiji, French Polynesia, Guam, New Caledonia, Papua New Guinea, Solomon Islands, Samoa, Timor Leste, Vanuatu.

## Australia

The population was estimated at 20.3 million in 2006. Over the period 2000–2005 life expectancy at birth was 80 years and infant mortality was five per thousand births. The population is 50.4% Protestant, 24.3% Roman Catholic and the rest non-Christian. In the year 2003 the birth rate was 13 per thousand and the death rate seven per thousand, a rate of natural increase of 0.6%. In 2005 the average woman had 1.8 children and if trends continue the population will be 25.6 million by the year 2050 (Wright 2006: 48). The capital city is Canberra with a population of 325,000 but the two biggest cities are Sydney (3.7 million) and Melbourne 3.2 million (1993 estimates). Like the USA, Australia has a federal structure, but because there is no supreme court each of the seven states can decide its own law. Australia is divided into the Capital Territory and seven states: South Australia, Victoria, Northern Territory, Tasmania, New South Wales, Western Australia and Queensland.

The Australian law was based on the 1861 British act. When activists began to think about liberalisation, as elsewhere they had to choose whether to work for legalisation through parliament or through the courts. Before legalisation, abortion was often performed by doctors for financial gain and with the agreement of the local police. In 1969 in Victoria, four members of the police force were convicted after abortionists were offered protection against prosecution for 10% of their fees (Wainer 1972). This raised interest in the possibility of change in the law as did the 1967 British act. South Australia was the first state to pass a liberal law in 1969. The wording was akin to that in Britain and allowed abortion when 'continuance of the pregnancy would involve greater risk to the life of the pregnant woman or greater risk of injury to the physical or mental health of the pregnant woman than if the pregnancy were terminated'. This wording had been used to support abortion on request in Britain.

In Victoria the law was changed through the courts. It was broadened by the case R v Davidson (1969) – also known as the Menhennitt ruling – where a State Supreme Court judge gave direction on the use of the word 'unlawfully' as used in the British 1861 act and copied into the legislation (see p.36). The judge tried to specify what was meant by 'unlawfully': 'I think that the accused must have honestly believed on reasonable grounds that the act done by him was necessary to preserve the woman from some serious danger.' He continued that the danger should not be only to the woman's life but also to her physical or mental health.

Northern Territory passed a liberalising law in 1973 (Paxman 1980). In New South Wales the law in operation from 1900 allowed abortion if the woman's life or health, mental or physical, was judged to be endangered by the pregnancy. In a trial in 1971, five people, including two doctors, were acquitted on charges of unlawfully terminating pregnancies. Mr Justice Levine expanded the term 'mental health' to include social and economic stress.

In Tasmania from 1925 to 2001 the law prohibited 'unlawful abortion'. In 2001 it passed a law similar to that of Southern Australia. In New South Wales two court rulings liberalised the law – the Levine ruling of 1971 and the Kirby ruling of 1994. Western Australia passed a law on 29 May 1998 which allowed abortion on request up to 20 weeks' gestation with the only condition being that the woman undergo counselling by a medical practitioner other than the one performing the operation.

Many have regarded Queensland as the most conservative of the states. For example, in 1977 it banned street assemblies. After anti-abortion groups had failed in an attempt to impose the existing law on a clinic in Brisbane an attempt was made to introduce a very conservative law. It would allow abortion only for rape or incest after police investigations. Rubella in the early stages of pregnancy, for example, would not have been sufficient grounds. A doctor who advised a woman to go to New South Wales for an abortion would be regarded as frustrating the objects of the act (section 19) and could be struck off the medical register. The bill was opposed by 3,000 women who defied the street assembly ban and was also opposed by the Australian Medical Association. In the event 19 members of the government crossed the floor to oppose the bill and secure its defeat (Francome 1984a: 152). In 2002 the Australian Capital Territory removed abortion from its penal code (Katzive 2007).

## New Zealand

The population was estimated at 4.1 million in 2006. Over the period 2000–2005 life expectancy at birth was 79 years and infant mortality was five per thousand births. The population is 52% Protestant, 15% Roman Catholic and 33% no religion or unspecified. In the year 2003 the birth rate was 14 per thousand and the death rate eight per thousand, a rate of natural increase of 0.6%. In 2005 the average woman had 2.0 children and if trends continue the population will be 4.8 million by the year 2050 (Wright 2006: 488). The capital city is Wellington with a population of 327,000 but the biggest city is Auckland with a population of 910,000 (1993 estimates).

The abortion law in New Zealand was also modelled on the British 1861 Offences Against the Person Act and was relatively restrictive. The number of therapeutic abortions in public hospitals more than quadrupled during the period 1969–1973. A crucial development was the setting up of the Auckland Medical Aid Centre in May 1974. This aimed to provide cheap abortions and though 80% of general practitioners had referred patients to it there were several attempts to close it (*Guardian* 24 October 1978). Opposition to a liberal abortion act was relatively strong and the Society for the Protection of the Unborn Child (SPUC) was formed in 1970 and by May 1975 was able to organise an 8,000-strong march on parliament. It was more extreme than the British equivalent and more like the absolutists in the USA.

The Royal Commission (1977) drew attention to the fact that it carried out more abortions than all the other public and private hospitals together. In 1975 one of its doctors, James Woolnough, was tried in the Supreme Court on twelve counts of using an instrument to procure abortions. The judge employed the same argument on the use of the word 'unlawfully' as had been employed in the earlier trial in South Australia. Woolnough was acquitted in a second trial after a hung jury and the law was effectively extended. However, a restrictive law was passed on 14 December 1977 and abortion was not even allowed in the case of fetal handicap. This law was unpopular and Facer (1978) reports a poll that showed only 15% approving the act and 66% disapproving. The Auckland centre closed immediately after the act came into effect and the number of abortions was reduced in the following year. The Sisters Overseas Service (SOS) arranged for women to fly to Australia but then the Auckland Centre reopened and by 1980 the rates of abortion were back to the level of 1976.

## Papua New Guinea

The population of Papua New Guinea was estimated to be 5.7 million in 2006. It gained its independence on 16 September 1975. Over the period 2000–2005 life expectancy at birth was 56 years. The population is 44% Protestant, 34% indigenous beliefs and 22% Roman Catholic. Jessica Redwood of Marie Stopes International commented (April 2007, personal communication) that in the country spirituality is tied to most actions, irrespective of official religions. People switch between denominations and 'traditional cultural beliefs are engrained within each person'. The country is the world's second biggest island and, because its population is disparate, a total of 850 languages are spoken. In the year 2003 the birth rate was 31 per thousand and the death rate eight per thousand, a rate of natural increase of 2.3%. In 2005 the average woman had 3.9 children and if trends continue the population will be 10.6 million by the year 2050 (Wright 2006: 488). The capital is Port Moresby with 174,000 inhabitants (1990 estimate).

There are many cultures within the country and a variety of patterns of relationship. Overall, researchers claim that the average age of first intercourse for both sexes is around 15 or 16 years. Observers report some strange beliefs which can affect the number of unwanted pregnancies, for example, many people believe pregnancy will not occur until couples have sex at least six times. Consequently this leads to people changing their partners frequently (Olivier Miller 2004 personal communication).

There is a variety of different patterns of sexuality amongst the Banaro: men have a virtual brother who is a kind of 'alter ego'. This special relationship is so strong that the men can have sex with each other's wives and this is not regarded as adultery. There is a strong sex divide and one observer commented: 'Women are valued as objects to be owned by men along with pigs and gardens.'

Abortion is illegal but the number seems to have been increasing. Consequently, one observer comments, 'It is not unusual to hear about young girls and older women inducing abortions.' These often lead to serious infections and even the death of the woman. The abortions are usually effected by herbs or inserting items into the vagina (Olivier Miller 2004 personal communication).

## Timor-Leste

In 2004 the national census revealed that the country had 923,000 people with men making up 50.9% of the population. Life expectancy was 49.5 years in 2004, an increase from 42.5 years in 1990. The maternal mortality rate was 660 per 100,000 live births, which is relatively high. The infant mortality rate in 2004 was 64, a reduction from 166 in 1990. Our local informant told us why she became involved in helping provide reproductive health services in the country: 'I felt compelled to work in reproductive health so as to help alleviate poverty and infant and maternal mortality in Timor-Leste.' She told us that the country gained its freedom from Indonesia and was placed under UN administration for two years before gaining full independence on 20 May 2004. We are advised that 'during the process of separation the health service was much damaged and reproductive health was not a great priority. The country has great reproductive health problems and at least 15 mothers die each week because of pregnancy related problems. The average woman has eight children, however, more than half of them die before they are five years old.'

There is little knowledge of modern forms of contraception, leading to our informant commenting that nine out of ten married women do not know about contraception and in addition: 'The majority of East Timorese have never seen a condom and do not know how to use it or what it is for.' The figures tend to support her, and the national census reveals that in 1990 one in five (20%) married women were using contraception but this figure fell to below one in ten (9%) in 2004. Things may be changing and condoms are now sold in the capital, Dili. The cost of condoms is high relative to local income; in 2007 the Ministry of Health and UNFPA began providing free condoms in community health centres. Marie Stopes International arrived in the country in 2006 and began its outreach programme in April 2007.

Abortion is illegal except to save the life of the woman. Consequently many of the abortions are carried out clandestinely. Our respondent commented: 'Traditional methods of abortion are used but they are shrouded in secrecy. Illegal abortion frequently causes a need for post-abortion care.'

## Vanuatu

The country consists of 12 major and 60 smaller islands in the Pacific Ocean and the population was estimated at 209,000 in 2006. Over the period 2000–2005 life expectancy at birth was 68 years. The population is 56% Protestant, 15% Roman Catholic, 8% indigenous beliefs, 6% Seventh Day Adventist and 16% other. In the year 2003 the birth rate was 26 per thousand and the death rate eight per thousand, a rate of natural increase of 1.8%. In 2005 the average woman had 3.9 children and if trends continue the population will be 375,000 by the year 2050 (Wright 2006: 48). The capital is Port Villa with a population of 19,000 (1989 estimate).

In 2005 the death of three young babies, possibly unnecessarily, led to concerns that many women were not getting the support they needed. Mrs Merilyn Tahi of the Women's Crisis Centre called upon the government to revise the abortion law. She pointed out that many women went abroad for their operations and that it could be only the richer women who had the resources (Radio Vanuatu 11 May).

## Conclusion

The area has undergone rapid change. In the twentieth century Margaret Mead's famous book *Coming of Age in Samoa* was a study of a primitive people who had a relaxed attitude towards sex from which she felt Americans could learn. When towards the end of the century the Samoans beat the Welsh at rugby football we realised that the country had 'come into' the modern world in a short time. There is still poverty and illiteracy amongst the poor countries of the area. However, the closeness of these countries to

Australia and New Zealand raises their awareness of the wealth towards which they might aspire, as well as allowing them to observe the advantages of developed societies. For this reason we may expect rapid change to continue in the area.

# NORTH AMERICA

*In the absence of any law, about 60% of minors say one or both parents are aware that they are having abortions. The proportion is higher among younger teenagers, reaching as high as 90% of those under age 14.*

**Henshaw and Kost 1992**

The birth rate for North America has largely remained constant at 2.0 children per woman. The rate dropped slightly to 1.9 children per woman during 1990–1995 but otherwise has been remarkably stable (Wright 2006: 483).

## Canada

In 2006 the population was 31.6 million (Statistics Canada 2007a). The fertility rate in 2005 was 1.5 children per woman; this rate had remained stable for the previous ten years. The majority of the Canadian population identify themselves as either Roman Catholic (43%) or Protestant (35%) while 16% claim no religious affiliation. Muslims, Hindus, Sikhs, Buddhists and Jews each constitute approximately 1–2% of the population (Statistics Canada 2003). The population is concentrated in the southern part of the country with over 80% living in urban areas. Over 60% of the population live in just two provinces, Ontario and Quebec. Alberta and the territory of Nunavut are the only two regions where the natural population increase is rising with births exceeding deaths. The birth rate in Nunavut is twice the national average (Statistics Canada 2006).

From 1869, abortion providers were liable to life imprisonment while any woman inducing her own abortion could be sentenced to seven years' imprisonment (Childbirth by Choice Trust 1998). In 1892 the government, influenced by the passage of restrictive US laws on birth control, prohibited the sale, advertisement and dissemination of contraceptives and abortifacients in the Criminal Code (McLaren and McLaren 1997). In 1969 the government, under the leadership of its prime minister Pierre Trudeau, reformed the Criminal Code. It decriminalised contraception and legalised abortion where continuation of the pregnancy 'would or would be likely to' endanger the life or health of the pregnant woman. Only a hospital-based 'therapeutic abortion committee' composed of three to five physicians could determine on a case-by-case basis if an abortion were necessary. Few hospitals established these committees and those that did were located primarily in urban centres. There were also weaknesses in the system as not all doctors were willing to serve in the abortion process and as the definition of 'health' varied tremendously. Although the law was restrictive, the number of abortions increased from 11,000 in 1970 to 43,000 in 1973 (Francome 1984a: 154). The opposition of pro-choice feminists, physicians and activists to the restrictions of the 1969 law coalesced around Henry Morgentaler, a Montreal physician. Morgentaler repeatedly broke the law by terminating pregnancies in the abortion clinics he established in Montreal, Toronto and Winnipeg. After several court battles, the Supreme Court struck down the abortion law in 1988 (Brodie et al. 1992; Dunphy 1996). The majority opinion held that the 1969 law violated a woman's right to 'life, liberty and security of person' under the Canadian Charter of Rights and Freedoms. A year later, the Court ruled in Tremblay vs. Daigle that there was no legal precedent for fetal personhood or for a father's right over the fetus. The government introduced a bill in 1990 intending to criminalise abortion but it failed in the Senate (Dickens 1991). Since the Supreme Court decision there has been no federal law regulating abortion in Canada (Rodgers 2006); it seems Canada is the only country in the world with no abortion law.

After the passage of the 1969 law, the rate of legal therapeutic abortions climbed steadily, levelling off in 1978 (Muldoon 1991). Most recent data reveal that in 2003, 103,600 legal abortions were performed. This was a slight decrease from 2002 (Statistics Canada 2006). Of these abortions, 56,100 were performed in public sector hospitals and

47,500 were performed in clinics operating in the public or private sector (Statistics Canada 2007b). Since 1997 the abortion rate for women aged 15–19 years has declined steadily from 18.4 per thousand women to 14.5 per thousand women in 2003. The birth rate for teenage women in 2003 was 12.1 births per thousand women, a significant reduction from the 1997 rate of 16.8 births per thousand women. Abortion in Canada is now most common among women in their twenties and this group accounted for 53% of all women who had abortions in 2003 (Statistics Canada 2006).

The illegality of abortion forced women to self-abort or to seek out medical practitioners – or even unqualified persons – who were willing to perform clandestine abortions. While most women survived, many died from subsequent infections. By the 1960s, abortion was a leading cause of maternal death in some provinces. Owing to the restrictive conditions of the 1969 law, illegal abortions were estimated at 100,000 a year. Those who could afford to, travelled for the procedure to countries such as Sweden, Japan, Great Britain and the USA where legal abortion was more accessible (Badgley et al. 1977; Pelrine 1972). Since 1988, abortion has been not only legal but also fully funded as a medically necessary service under the Canada Health Act. This act requires that medically necessary services be accessible, portable, universal, comprehensive and publicly administered (Health Canada 2002). Therefore, any restrictions on access to abortions technically violate the terms of the act. Nevertheless, access is grossly uneven across the country because of the absence of abortion services in some areas, such as in the province of Prince Edward Island. In other instances, access is uneven owing to differences in provincial health insurance plans to fund abortions, the refusal of some provinces to exclude abortion from reciprocal billing agreements, and the imposition of termination committees in some hospitals. For example, the province of New Brunswick pays for abortions only if they are approved by two obstetricians or gynaecologists and are performed in a hospital. Moreover, abortions are not always fully funded. The courts have ruled recently that such impediments violate women's rights under the Canadian Charter of Rights and Freedoms and the terms of the Canada Health Act (Bourque 2006; CBC 2004; Chiarelli 2004; Palley 2006; Rodgers 2006). The reduction in abortion services in public sector hospitals has similarly contributed to uneven access to abortion. Hospitals sometimes place obstacles in the way of women trying to obtain an abortion; hospital employees may not be able to provide women with information about alternative abortion services; and physicians and hospital employees may deny women access by refusing information and referrals, or by referring women to anti-choice agencies (Shaw 2007). Finally, access is uneven because clinics operating in the private sector in a non-profit or for-profit capacity are concentrated in major cities. Consequently, travel to access abortion services is a necessity for some young women, poor women and for women living in rural and eastern Canada (Eggertson 2001; McCracken 2002). As of April 2007, RU-486 has not received Health Canada approval. Some doctors, however, prescribe a combination of misoprostol and methotrexate to induce a medical abortion within the first seven weeks of pregnancy. Surgical abortion remains the most popular method of abortion in Canada.

## Specific events in Canada

The 1969 law galvanised emerging feminist groups to organise a march to the capital of Ottawa in an 'abortion caravan' for a Mother's Day protest in May 1970. Once there, the women chained themselves to the Visitors' Gallery in Parliament and dumped a coffin filled with coat hangers (as a symbol of illegal abortion) on the grounds of the prime minister's residence.

In 1975, the Criminal Code was revised yet again to include a 'Morgentaler amendment' that prevented appeal courts from overturning jury verdicts as had occurred in the Morgentaler case.

A former politician, Joe Borowski, went on a hunger strike in 1981 to draw attention to the lack of protection for the unborn in the Charter of Rights and Freedoms. In 1992 the Toronto Morgentaler Clinic was firebombed, signalling an escalation in anti-abortion activity. During the 1990s, three doctors who performed abortions in Manitoba, Ontario and British Columbia were shot and wounded. The main suspect is James Kopp, a self-professed anti-abortionist who is currently on trial in the USA for the murder of an American doctor who performed abortions. In the lead-up to the federal election of 2004, one member of the Conservative party made headlines when he indicated that he would support limits on women's access to abortion. The comment ignited debate about abortion (Wente 2004). Since the minority Conservative government was elected in 2006, two private members have introduced anti-abortion measures to parliament. Bill C-291 is intended to criminalise the causation of injury or death of a child before or during its birth. Bill C-338 would jail and/or fine those performing abortions after 20 weeks.

Polls show that the majority of Canadians support safeguarding access to abortion. Groups favouring the former position include: Canadians for Choice, which is engaged in research; Medical Students for Choice, which promotes the teaching of abortion procedures in medical education; Action Canada for Population and Development, which campaigns at a national and international political level for women's reproductive rights; Abortion Rights Coalition of Canada, which is engaged in research and advocacy work emphasising the issue of abortion rights in Canada; and the National Abortion Federation in Canada, which supports, trains and protects abortion providers.

A minority wish to recriminalise abortion or to place limitations on access to abortion (CBC 1998). Groups which favour the latter position include Realistic Equal and Active for Life (REAL) and Women and Campaign for Life Coalition, both of which endorse 'pro-life' candidates running for election. Crisis Pregnancy Centers counsel women against abortion as an option (Johansen 2004). Canadian Physicians for Life holds that human life begins at conception and supports conscience clauses to protect doctors who do not wish to provide abortions. Focus on the Family Canada, with ties to its parent organisation in the USA, lobbies for the nuclear family and is opposed to gay marriage, premarital sex and abortion:

It is expected that the majority of Canadians will resist any attempt to criminalize abortion or to place limitations on access to it. However, the current controversy over the positive and negative aspects of public vs. private health care in Canada will increasingly have an impact on the delivery of abortion services. Public sector hospitals may outsource abortion services to private sector non-profit abortion clinics while private sector for-profit abortion clinics might increase in number. It is anticipated that there will be heightened legal wrangling between federal and provincial powers in regard to abortion coverage leading to more court challenges. If abortion remains a medically necessary service under the Canada Health Act it is likely that women paying for and/or travelling to access abortion procedures will continue to seek financial reimbursement for costs incurred. To prevent women from having abortions, groups favouring the criminalization of abortion or the placement of limitations on access might push to remove abortion as a medically necessary service from the Canada Health Act, fund more CPCs as a counterweight to public and private sector abortion services and make inroads with those Members of Parliament, who, regardless of political affiliation, do not support abortion. Some women's groups and medical bodies will demand that Health Canada approve RU-486; if successful, it will be opposed by groups opposing abortion. Finally, the global growth in fetal screening may result in increases in abortion as a means of sex selection or for the purposes of eliminating genetic abnormalities (Christabelle Sethna and Marion Doull, University of Ottawa, personal communication).

## United States of America

The population was estimated at 298.4 million in 2006. Over the period 2000–2005 life expectancy at birth was 77 years and the infant mortality rate seven per thousand births. Fifty-two per cent are Protestant, 24% Roman Catholic, 10% have no religion, 2% are Mormon, 1% Jewish and 10% other. In 2003 the birth rate was 14 per thousand and the death rate eight per thousand, a rate of natural increase of 0.6%. In 2005 the fertility rate was 2.0 children and if current rates persist the population will be 408.7 million by the year 2050 (Wright 2006: 483, 699).

Individual states made abortion illegal in the nineteenth century. The first person to systematically argue for its legalisation was William Robinson, the editor of the journal *Critic and Guide*, in 1913. He called for legalisation of abortion in the early stages of pregnancy but disagreed with the German Professor Kocks who argued for legalisation throughout pregnancy (Francome 1984a: 75). Robinson felt, however, that abortion should be performed only sparingly and this led him to express criticism of some of the young people of his day. He argued for reform of the laws and his position was supported by a woman's group which formed the Association for the Reform of the Abortion Laws in 1932 (Taussig 1936: 426). This group aimed to broaden the grounds for abortion to include cases of rape, seduction, infirmity, likely handicap, destitution and divorce. Such calls were likely to be unsuccessful in a society when the doctors' main medical association did not even accept contraception until 1937 (Francome 1984a: 76).

At the outbreak of the Second World War abortion was illegal in every state except Mississippi but in some states there were legal exemptions. In six states there were no legal exemptions. In 39 states abortion was legal to save the life of the woman and in a further three states and the District of Columbia abortion was also allowed for the health of the woman. In Mississippi alone the operation was legal at the discretion of the medical practitioner (Birkett 1939: 165).

## Changing the law

In the post-war years the early pressure was for the abortion law to be extended, but not as far as to allow abortion on request. In December 1959 the America Law Institute revealed its model bill which would legalise abortion if continuation would 'gravely impair the physical or mental health of the mother' for rape or incest and for fetal abnormality. In 1967 the American Medical Association gave support for change in the law and this led to bills being passed. The first bill passed was in Colorado in 1967; California and North Carolina followed shortly afterwards. In 1968 Georgia and Maryland liberalised their laws and in 1969 were followed by Arkansas, Kansas,

Delaware, Oregon and New Mexico. The first state to pass a law giving women abortion on request was Hawaii in 1970, but this law required the woman to be a resident of the state. By this time, rich women could obtain legal abortions in Britain, and it was the legalisation of abortion on request up to 24 weeks in New York State which first gave US women the right to legal abortion on request in their own country.

In 1972 the Massachusetts law banning contraception for single people was overturned by the Supreme Court on the grounds of privacy. This was one of the factors which paved the way for the Supreme Court decision of 22 January 1973 which made all abortion laws in the USA unconstitutional. The decision in Roe vs. Wade divided pregnancy into trimesters. In the first trimester, abortion was legal on the grounds of privacy and the decision left to the woman and her attending physician. From the second trimester, however, the interests of the state in promoting the health of the woman became of increased importance and so states were free to regulate abortion procedures in ways that were reasonably related to maternal health. Once fetal viability had been reached, a state could proscribe abortion in accordance with its interest in the potential human life except when it was necessary to preserve the life or health of the woman (Osofsky and Osofsky 1973).

During the 1970s and 1980s, the Supreme Court found that many states had introduced restrictions which were unconstitutional under Roe vs. Wade. In 1992, in the case of Planned Parenthood of Southeastern Pennsylvania vs. Casey, it relaxed the standards that restrictions have to meet in order to be constitutional. In that case, it held that although women still have the right to terminate a pregnancy as established by Roe vs. Wade, restrictions are permissible as long as they do not constitute an 'undue burden' on women, that is, they do not have the purpose or effect of placing a substantial obstacle in the path of a woman seeking an abortion. Although federal constitutional protection of abortion rights has been limited by this and other decisions, a number of state constitutions contain stronger protections. According to the Center for Reproductive Rights, the highest courts of ten states have interpreted their state constitutions to provide explicit protection to abortion rights. Six other states have strong statutory protection for the right to have an abortion and, according to the Center, seven others are unlikely to ban abortion if Roe vs. Wade were overruled (2004). Nevertheless, even where abortion is considered a basic right by the courts, restrictions that block some women from access to abortion services are common. Following are the major restrictions that are now in effect in some or all states.

### Medicaid coverage unavailable for abortion services

In 1977, Congress eliminated coverage of most abortions under the National Health Insurance Plan for Poor Families and also the in the National Plan for Poor Families' Health in 1980, the Supreme Court held that the government has no constitutional responsibility to provide funds for medically necessary abortions. Currently the 'Hyde amendment' prohibits federal payment for abortions other than those for pregnancies caused by rape or incest or those necessary to save the woman's life. Nevertheless, some states continue to pay for most medically necessary abortions under their Medicaid programmes without the benefit of federal funding. In most cases, coverage is a result of a court order based on the state constitution (as in Alaska, Arizona, California, Connecticut, Illinois, Massachusetts, Minnesota, Montana, New Jersey, New Mexico, Oregon, Vermont and West Virginia). In several of these states, however, Medicaid reimbursement is difficult to obtain despite the court order. Four states cover abortion voluntarily: these are Hawaii, Maryland, New York and Washington (Guttmacher Institute 2006). Studies of the effect of Medicaid funding have found that a significant number of women who would have had abortions with Medicaid coverage instead continue their pregnancies when they are obliged to pay the abortion charges out of pocket. Cook et al. (1999) examined abortion and birth rates in North Carolina, where the legislature created a special fund to pay for abortions for poor women. Several times, the fund was exhausted before the end of the fiscal year, so that financial support was unavailable to women whose pregnancies occurred after that point in the year before the next year's funding became available. The analysis found that about one-third of the women who would have had abortions when support was available instead carried their pregnancies to term when the abortion fund was unavailable. Similarly, Trussell et al. (1980) in Michigan, Ohio and Georgia found that 18–22% of women who would have had abortions continued their pregnancies after Medicaid funding was cut off, and Chrissman et al. (1980) in Texas found that 35% of women did so. One can assume that the women who are unable to overcome the barrier posed by lack of financial support for the abortion are those with the fewest financial resources. These are also likely to be women who are not in a favourable position to take responsibility for the care and support of children. Women with borderline motivation to prevent childbirth may also be affected by lack of financial support for abortion.

## Parental notification or consent for minors

In Bellotti vs. Baird (1979) and in other decisions, the Supreme Court held that unemancipated minors could be required to notify one or both parents or obtain their consent before obtaining an abortion, provided that an alternative is available to prevent parents from having an absolute ability to block the abortion. In most cases, the alternative is access to a judge, who must grant the abortion request if the minor is mature enough to make an informed decision or if the abortion is in the minor's best interest. As of 2006, 22 states require that minors obtain the consent of one or both parents and 13 that one or both parents be notified. All of these states provide for a judicial bypass and six also have provision for notice or consent of another adult relative (Guttmacher Institute 2006). Although the asserted purpose of these laws is to encourage minors to consult their parents before having an abortion, there is little evidence that this has been accomplished where judicial bypass is available. One study comparing the proportion of minors who consulted parents in Minnesota, where such a requirement was in effect, with Wisconsin, where there was no such requirement, found little difference in the proportion of minors whose parents knew about their abortions (Blum et al. 1987). In the absence of such a legal requirement, about 60% of minors say one or both parents are aware of their abortions. The proportion is higher among younger teenagers, reaching as high as 90% of those under the age of 14 (Henshaw and Kost 1992). One immediate effect of these regulations, however, is that minors travel to neighbouring states to avoid parental involvement requirements or to states with less stringent requirements. A study of the effect of a Massachusetts parental consent regulation found that the number of Massachusetts minors having abortions in Rhode Island, New Hampshire, and other states rose significantly but there was little change in the total number of minors having abortions or giving birth when out-of-state services were taken into account (Cartoof and Klerman 1986).

Similarly, studies in Mississippi and Missouri found increases in the number of minors obtaining abortion services in other states (Henshaw 1995). Another possible effect of parental involvement regulations is that minors would continue more of their pregnancies, either because they consulted parents who favoured continuation of the pregnancy or because they delayed dealing with the pregnancy to the point where abortion was no longer possible. Studies in Massachusetts and Mississippi found little increase in the birth rates to minors, suggesting that any such effect would be small (Cartoof and Klerman 1986; Henshaw 1995). One study that took age into account found that among women who conceived at the age of 17, a larger proportion gave birth after a parental notice regulation came into effect in Texas (Joyce et al. 2006). Overall, however, the effect is small.

Another effect of these regulations is to delay abortions. Statistics from Minnesota and Mississippi show that parental involvement regulations increase the proportion of minors whose abortions are past 12 weeks by about one-fifth (Rogers et al. 1991; Henshaw 1995). There was a similar increase in Missouri. Since fewer than half of minors wish to avoid involving their parents, the impact on these minors is greater than the overall figures would suggest. Delay could be caused by reluctance of the minors to go to court or involve their parents, the wait to see a judge, and the time required to arrange for travel to other states. The study in Texas also found that women who were nearly 18 years old delayed their abortion until their eighteenth birthday, resulting in a raised number of later abortions among women exactly 18 years old (Joyce et al. 2006). Some proponents of parental involvement requirements believe that they prevent teenage pregnancy, either by reducing sexual activity or by causing minors to use contraception more conscientiously. Opponents of parental involvement requirements have argued that they harm minors in some cases, especially where there is parental abuse or family conflict. No systematic research has examined this question. A survey of minors having abortions in states without parental involvement requirements found that conflict occurred when parents found out about the abortion without having been told by the pregnant girl. Severe consequences resulted in a small proportion of these cases, including the minor suffering physical violence and being forced to leave home. In sum, parental involvement requirements cause delay and out-of-state travel, and result in an unknown level of family conflict that is harmful to the minors. In a few cases, they may result in families causing minors to continue unwanted pregnancies. The benefits of increased parental support and pregnancy prevention are small or non-existent. Whereas opinion polls show support for parental involvement regulations, the public has rejected such regulations in referendums in California and Oregon and narrowly approved them in Colorado and Florida.

### State-mandated counselling and waiting periods

An increasing number of states, 29 as of 2006, require that women receive state-directed counselling, that is, that they be given certain specific information before an abortion can be performed. This information frequently includes the risks of abortion and childbirth, a description of fetal development, the assistance available to women for prenatal care, childbirth and infant care, and a list of agencies that provide information or services designed to help women carry their pregnancies to term. Three states require that women be told that having an abortion may increase the risk of breast cancer, even though medical authorities are in agreement that no such relationship exists. Four states require that women be told that a fetus at 20 weeks or more may feel pain and be offered anaesthesia for the fetus, and three require that women be given information on the possible psychological effects of abortion. A majority of the states require that the state-mandated counselling must take place a specified number of hours, usually 24, before the abortion can be performed. Six states require that the information be delivered in person, which means that in most cases the woman must make two trips to the abortion facility.

The Supreme Court held, in 1983 in City of Akron vs. Akron Center for Reproductive Health, that state-directed counselling and waiting period requirements are unconstitutional and reaffirmed this decision with respect to counselling in 1986 in Thornburgh vs. American College of Obstetricians and Gynecologists, Pennsylvania Section. Nevertheless, it overruled these decisions in Pennsylvania vs. Casey in 1992, when it found that required counselling and waiting periods did not violate the new 'undue burden' criterion.

Although proponents of these requirements say they are needed to help women make informed decisions, the implicit purpose is to discourage abortion. Evidence for this is that no similar requirements apply to women seeking prenatal care, though the decision to continue a pregnancy carries more risk and responsibility than the decision to terminate a pregnancy. Abortion providers have found that the required counselling and waiting periods have little effect on women's abortion decisions, although they object in principle to the assumption that women need special constraints when making important decisions and that the state can override the judgement of medical professionals about the information needed by their patients. It is not clear whether the required counselling succeeds in evoking guilt in women having abortions. The two-trip requirement, however, may be a significant burden and prevent some women from obtaining desired abortion services. A study of abortion statistics from Mississippi and neighbouring states found that approximately 11% of the women who would have had abortions were prevented from doing so by a two-trip requirement. In addition, many women went to other states to avoid the requirement, and abortions were delayed on average (Joyce et al. 2006).

In summary, the counselling and waiting period requirements appear to serve little purpose except to act as a barrier to services and possibly to further stigmatise abortion.

### Clinic licensing and other restrictions on abortion facilities

In the 1960s, abortion was considered a dangerous procedure that should be performed in hospitals. After the law was liberalised in New York in 1970, hospitals were unable to meet the demand, so clinics were established that used a simpler and safer procedure, vacuum aspiration. Studies in the 1970s demonstrated that first-trimester and early second-trimester abortions in clinics are as safe as those performed in hospitals. In the Akron decision (see above) and in Planned Parenthood of Kansas City, Missouri vs. Ashcroft (1983), the Supreme Court held that states could not require that all second-trimester abortions be performed in hospitals. However, laws requiring that clinics be licensed and meet strict standards for the facility and staff have generally not been found to be unconstitutional. Despite the excellent safety record of abortion clinics, a number of states have recently imposed burdensome licensing requirements. In many cases, clinics must meet surgical standards which often approach the standards of hospitals. For example, the standards specify the amount of air flow, the size of corridors, the number and location of toilets and dressing areas for staff, and the like. There have been no studies to show that such measures improve the safety of abortions or that they prevent deaths or complications.

## Protection of access to clinic entrances

In the mid-1980s, anti-abortion protests became increasingly violent and destructive. Bombings, arson, vandalism, blockades and violent protests were common. In 1994, the federal government enacted the Freedom of Access to Clinic Entrances Act, which prohibits the use of force or physical obstruction to interfere with someone entering a reproductive health care facility. This act, together with other factors such as the increasing political success of anti-abortion groups, is credited with a reduction in clinic violence. In addition to the federal law, some 13 states and the District of Columbia prohibit certain anti-abortion activities directed at abortion providers such as blocking of clinic entrances and intimidating staff. Three states and several municipalities have protected 'bubble zones', regions of a specified number of feet around a person within a certain distance of a clinic that cannot be entered by a protester without the person's consent.

## Other abortion-related policies

State laws on a number of other issues affect abortion providers and access to abortion services. Three states prohibit private health insurance from covering abortion services except in a rider with an additional charge, and several states prohibit health insurance for public employees from covering abortion. Several states require that abortions be performed by physicians. These laws can prevent mid-level practitioners from performing simple abortions, even with the medication mifepristone. Abortion services may not be performed in any public facilities, including state medical school hospitals, in several states. Requirements for the disposal of fetal remains increase providers' costs in some states.

## Policy trends

Recent changes in the make-up of the Supreme Court may result in relaxation of the limits on the extent to which abortion can be restricted. While it is possible that the Roe vs. Wade decision could be reversed, the predominant thinking is that the Court will permit more severe restrictions without entirely overruling Roe vs. Wade. However, it is difficult to predict how new justices will decide issues they have not previously encountered.

# The practice of legal abortion

Currently there are about 1.3 million abortions a year in the USA, a rate of about 21 abortions per thousand women aged 15–44 (Finer and Henshaw 2006). That is, each year about 2% of women of childbearing age have an abortion. Abortion rates are relatively high in large metropolitan areas and low in small towns and rural areas. This may be in part because of greater availability of abortion services in metropolitan areas. Abortion rates are high among black women (57 per thousand) and Hispanic women (31 per thousand) in comparison with non-Hispanic white women (12 per thousand) (Ventura 2004). Other groups with especially high abortion rates are women aged 18–24, never-married women, cohabiting women, and those with low income and eligible for Medicaid health insurance (Jones et al. 2002). The abortion rate has been falling slowly in recent years, mainly because of a reduction among teenagers and a decrease in the proportion of unintended pregnancies ending in abortion. Going against the overall trend are increasing unintended pregnancy and abortion rates among women whose income is below 200% of the federal poverty standard and among cohabiting women (Finer and Henshaw 2006). Prenatal screening, followed by abortion when necessary, has allowed couples to avoid the birth of children with congenital abnormalities. The result is a marked decrease in the number of such births. The number of children born in 2001 with Down syndrome was 3,654, about half the number of 7,262 that would be expected in the absence of screening (Egan et al. 2004). About 50% of women choose to continue pregnancies when abnormalities are identified; for some of those who end such pregnancies, the birth of a disabled child would be devastating psychologically, socially and economically.

## Conclusion

The overall figures show that all groups in the USA have abortion rates higher than in comparable European countries. For abortion rates to fall further in the USA, contraceptive usage needs to improve, which requires an improvement in the quality of sex education. The greatest effect might be felt if efforts were concentrated towards the most vulnerable groups such as those aged between 18 and 24 and the high risk ethnic groups.

# ILLEGAL ABORTION IN DEVELOPED COUNTRIES

*I DO DISLIKE A CERTAIN TYPE OF MODERN YOUNG
WOMAN WHO INDULGES PROMISCUOUSLY, USES
CONTRACEPTIVES RATHER RELUCTANTLY,
PREFERRING REPEAT ABORTIONS WHICH SHE
REGARDS AS LIGHTLY AS DOWNING DOWN A
COCKTAIL OR A GLASS OF WHISKY.*

**Dr William Robinson USA 1929**

W e have seen that there are two perspectives on the approach to sexuality. The first is to accept that people can make their own choices to enable them to make sound decisions based on quality sex education and to provide them with information about available methods of contraception. The other approach is to promote abstinence amongst those not married and to discourage contraception, with adoption being the alternative to those who bring a child into poor social conditions. Some people believe that in the Victorian era in the nineteenth century this latter situation pertained. Margaret Thatcher was one of those who praised Victorian values. It is therefore timely to remind ourselves of the problems of sexuality during this period. We will concentrate on Britain and the USA.

## The peculiar case of the safe period

We will be arguing that there were high numbers of abortions in the period up to around 1930 in part due to the absence of contraception and the misinformation that was prevalent concerning the safe period, causing women wishing to avoid pregnancy to have sexual intercourse at the most risky times in their cycle. One piece of research that led to this view was that of the German scientist, Thedor Bischoff who, in 1853, published his discovery about ova of the genital tract of bitches 'on heat' and concluded that women also must ovulate at the time of menstruation. Annie Besant in 1877 popularised this view and Marie Stopes continued the practice of quoting the wrong 'safe period' in her best-selling book *Married Love* (1918). This false information was obviously important to Roman Catholics who had received permission to use the safe period in 1853 and whose priests regularly quoted the erroneous information (Francome 1984b).

The Chief Rabbi cast doubt on this view of the safe period in 1917 because observant Jews had no intercourse until 12 days after the start of the menstrual period but did not have smaller families than non-observant Jews (Birth Rate Commission 1917). The first time people had reliable information was in 1925 when a study by Siegal was reported in Britain (Francome 1986: 22–3). He studied the wives of 320 German soldiers after their husbands had been home on leave for two to eight days. He found no conceptions after 21 days of the cycle and the Malthusians commented that his work 'proves beyond question that there is some truth in the doctrine of the safe period, and it also proves that this period comes later in the cycle than is commonly supposed' (Francome 1986). In the USA some books continued giving the wrong dates at least until 1928 and it was not until the early 1930s that the cycle became fully understood.

## Unsafe abortion in the USA

Abortion was legal throughout the USA in the early months of pregnancy until New York passed a law making it illegal in 1828. It seems that the authorities were concerned with the danger of the operation for women and that this was also the primary concern of other states. For example, the New Jersey law made it clear that it was trying to guard the health of women. In 1839 the well-known professor, Hugh Hodge, said that most abortions were 'to destroy the fruit of illicit pleasure' (Hodge 1854). At this time abortifacient pills were prominent. For example, on 4 Jan 1845 the *Boston Daily Times* carried an advertisement for Dr Peter's French Renovating Pills. It warned: 'Pregnant females should not use them as they invariably cause miscarriage.' Four years later it was reported that a Dr Sunot had developed an airtight cup from which the air could be removed and used on the 'lower body' to restore bleeding (Hollick 1849). Mohr, reviewing the evidence of the time, comments that by the 1850s and 1860s there was possibly one abortion for every five or six live births. As each woman had on average around six children it would seem that there were about as many abortions as there were women (1978: 50). Hodge (1854) was surprised that:

> Educated, refined and fashionable women whose moral character is in other respects without reproach, mothers who are devoted with an ardent and self denying affection to the children who already constitute their family, are perfectly indifferent respecting the fetus in utero.

In 1859 a committee of the Suffolk County Medical Association reported that abortion was common in all classes and in the following year Hale (1860) estimated that one in five pregnancies ended in abortion and that nine out of ten married women had attempted one. He said that in his own area of Chicago he had met women who had more than ten children and the same number of abortions (Francome 1986: 31).

Between 1860 and 1880, concern with women's health was a crucial factor in at least 40 statutes being passed to attempt to eliminate abortion. Horatio Storer, a key activist, published his concern that abortion was so dangerous that a woman procuring one could almost be looked upon as actually insane (1866: 15). He, like many subsequently, quoted results of a survey by Tardieu which reported that 34 abortions led to 22 deaths. Even 66 years later (1932) Parry felt it necessary to point out that Tardieu had had an unusual series. This kind of propaganda seems to have had little effect on the population who would have intimate knowledge of those who had had successful abortions. In May 1863 the *American Medical Times* carried an article about the 'wide and almost universal prevalence' of abortion and commented it was common in 'every grade of society' and that 'the religious equally entertain the belief that abortions may be practiced without a shadow of guilt' (Francome 1986: 34).

On 3 Nov 1870 the *New York Times* noted a British campaign against abortion, which we discuss below, and began to campaign against what it later called 'the evil of the age' (23 August 1871). The advertisements disappeared for a short time but then returned. Anthony Comstock was the man who took over the anti-sexuality mantle and persuaded Congress to attack both abortion and contraception. The second report of the Society for the Suppression of Vice (1876) said that 49 abortionists had been arrested and 39 of these had been convicted (Francome 1986: 36). The Comstock law did, however, contain an exception for abortions carried out by physicians of good standing and this may have been one of the factors leading to the suppression of unqualified operators and abortions being carried out by doctors.

In 1888 Pomeroy reported that the laws against abortion were a 'dead letter' and that they (abortions) flourished in the highest places. He said other countries talked of abortion as 'the American sin' and of advertisements which stated: 'Married ladies who have any reason to believe they are pregnant are particularly cautioned against using these pills as they will cause miscarriage.' In this year a series of articles appeared in the medical literature in support of contraception. Pope said doctors faced requests almost daily and that the use of the condom could lessen the death rate of both women and children. However, there was not widespread availability of contraception to reduce abortion rates and in 1896 abortion was sufficiently visible that the *Boston Medical and Surgical Journal* carried an article asking why it should be so common and stated that abortion advertisements were 'a source of danger to the innocent and uninstructed' (p. 541). In the 1890s some doctors were estimating that the USA had 2 million abortions a year (Gordon 1977: 53).

In 1906 another article appeared in favour of contraception when Jacobi, an eminent New York doctor, said it was no use telling a woman with syphilis she should not become pregnant without telling her how to avoid it: she would otherwise return a few months later and the doctor would empty her uterus but leave her in the same situation (Francome 1986: 39). The leading pro-choice activist during the early twentieth century was William Robinson. In his journal the *Critic and Guide* (January 1906), he gave advice to young medical practitioners. He told them that they would be asked to carry out abortions, commenting:

> An abortionist, who is aseptic and not too clumsy, can enjoy a lucrative practice with very
> few deaths and the man who refuses to perform abortions will lose a good deal of practice
> and make enemies of many influential persons (Francome 1986).

In this year Dr Hunter of Louisville carried out research into the practice of abortion by writing to 100 doctors. He calculated from the responses that in the USA there were over 100,000 abortions and 6,000 deaths each year (Medical Age March 1906). Other research was carried out by Taussig (1910). He studied 348 women who had been pregnant at least once. Of these, 201 reported they had had a total of 371 spontaneous or induced abortions. This is an average of over one per woman despite the fact that Taussig commented: 'It is always difficult to obtain a confession of such a criminal act from a patient.' He proposed that at least half these abortions were induced and reported that abortion is found 'in all classes, in all countries'. He believed abortion was increasing because antiseptic procedures were making it safer. Overall he estimated 80,000 illegal abortions in New York and 8,000–10,000 in Chicago.

In 1909 Robinson also stated that the number of abortions was high and two years later said that up to a quarter of doctors were regularly performing them (Francome 1986: 40). He believed that the number could be reduced:

> when the good moral, Christian people of our land look upon the maiden 'who loves not
> wisely but too well' with more charity and pity … then will the evils of abortion rapidly
> decline … let us recognize that bearing a child out of wedlock is not incompatible with
> true repentance and a future of honor.

In 1911 Robinson 'conservatively' estimated that there were one million abortions a year in the USA. This is half that of the estimates of some doctors in the 1890s. By 1917 Robinson had increased his estimate of the number of doctors performing abortions to 75% performing at some time or other (Francome 1986).

In the inter-war years the growth of contraception may at first have reduced the number of abortions. An anonymous survey of doctors known to have performed abortions estimates there were 550,000 abortions a year. This is well below the figure predicted earlier. One doctor reported he had carried out 18,000 abortions at $50 each and the author noted there were virtually no prosecutions and that the public supported the practice. He reported that when he saw a doctor driving by someone said that he was the leading abortionist in town; this was not a critical statement but as one would say in an offhand way, 'There's the Brooklyn Bridge' (Francome 1986: 42). In 1924 Ettie Arout was quoted in the *Critic and Guide* that as the result of suppression of contraception, abortions were widespread: 'Educated married women told me quite frankly that they had two or more abortions regularly every year, that they experienced no difficulty in securing efficient and economical service in this way.' Margaret Sanger told in her autobiography that ideas of what to do with an unwanted pregnancy were passed from mouth to mouth. She gave examples of herb teas, turpentine, rolling downstairs, inserting slippery elm and knitting needles. Other women visited local operators: 'On Saturday nights I have seen groups of from fifty to one hundred with their shawls over their heads waiting outside the office of the five dollar abortionist' (1938: 89).

One of the reasons for high abortion rates in the USA was the continued suppression of birth control. While in Britain birth control was effectively legalised in 1877, in the USA as late as 1935 the *Brooklyn Eagle* (6 January) reported that nine books and magazines largely dealing with birth control were banned from entry to the USA. It was not until 1937 that the medical profession endorsed contraception in the USA. The actual number of abortions in the inter-war years is a matter of debate. Robinson had been estimating 2 million a year. This he increased to 3 million in 1929 (*Critic and Guide*: 53). Margaret Sanger proposed the lower figure but commented in *New Generation* April 1935:

> It is the opinion of competent medical observers during the last twenty-five years that there are more criminal abortions in the USA than any other country in the world. The total of abortions, which does not include the number of those brought about by drugs or by instruments used by the pregnant woman herself, has been estimated to top two million a year.

Rongy (1933) also suggested 2 million abortions a year and the examples of individual women suggest that in the absence of contraception many women were having surprisingly high numbers. In 1933 the Critic and Guide told of a Dr Kahn who had investigated a perforated uterus and was told the woman had had seven abortions in two years. Later the journal told of a married 17-year-old who had had four abortions in one year. It would be almost impossible to find such a high incidence in modern-day USA. The 'modern young woman' quoted at the beginning of this chapter had had three abortions and was asking for a fourth (Francome 1984b: 75). In his second book, Taussig (1936) quoted the work of Dr Kopp, who investigated the records of 10,000 women at a birth control clinic. Just over half reported a total of 11,172 abortions of which 3,165 were spontaneous. Overall, one in five pregnancies ended in induced abortion. The higher number of pregnancies was a factor in the high number of abortions and Kopp's figures showed that for married women only 4% of first pregnancies were aborted compared with 28% of fourth pregnancies and 48% of the ninth or subsequent. In 1942 Alan Guttmacher quoted the New York Prosecutor that there were 100,000–250,000 abortions each year in the city alone (*New York Times* 31 January 1942).

After the Second World War estimates of the number of abortions were much lower. At a conference on abortion in 1957, Calderone suggested the figure could range from as low as 200,000 to as high as 1.2 million. Even the higher level is well below the 3 million predicted in the early 1930s. Subsequently it was the figure of one million that was most often quoted. In the period after the Second World War until 1970, although abortions were restricted in all states, illegal abortions were common. Women with resources and connections were able to obtain relatively safe abortions from physicians. Most of these abortions were performed illegally, but some women were able to have their pregnancies terminated in hospitals by convincing psychiatrists and hospital committees that the pregnancy posed a danger of suicide. Other women went to Puerto Rico where abortion was strictly illegal but nevertheless available. After April 27 1968 others could go to Britain for an abortion. Women without resources used primitive methods such as inserting an object into their uterus or going to an individual without medical training. Many serious complications and even deaths resulted.

A number of studies have tried to estimate the number of abortions that took place annually before 1970. A study based on the change in the birth rate in New York City after 1970 concluded that 70% of the legal abortions in 1971 replaced abortions that would have taken place anyway illegally. From a survey in North Carolina in 1967, researchers estimated that 829,000 abortions were occurring in the country as a whole, which is about 80% of the number of legal abortions that occurred in 1975, when legal abortion services were available in all states (Abernathy et al. 1970). The change in the number of births nationally suggests that roughly 600,000 abortions would have occurred without legalisation (Levine et al. 1999).

In the USA as well as in other countries, legalised abortion reduced mortality from induced abortion (Tietze et al. 1972). Over the decade from 1958 to 1967, more than 3,400 women died from induced abortion, almost all from illegal abortion (Hilgers and O'Hare 1981). The number of abortion deaths rose during the 1950s and reached at least 430 in 1961, then declined during the 1960s partly because more physicians became willing to terminate pregnancies. Legalisation of abortion resulted in a sharp fall in the number of deaths, from about 251 in 1966 to 14 in 1976, a reduction of 94%. In recent years, the number of deaths has ranged between four and 12 per year according to the Centers for Disease Control and Prevention (Strauss et al. 2004).

To the extent that legal abortion replaced childbirth, it also reduced maternal deaths because it was safer than continued pregnancy and delivery. During the period 1991–1999, mortality associated with live birth was 7.1 deaths per 100,000 live births (excluding deaths from miscarriage and ectopic pregnancy, which might not be prevented by abortion), compared with 0.6 deaths per 100,000 induced abortions (Grimes 1999). One researcher calculated that between 1970 and 1980, in the order of 1,500 women's lives were saved by the substitution of unwanted and mistimed births and illegal abortions by legal abortions. The saving might have been greater since, after legalisation of abortion, many more women with serious medical conditions were able to terminate potentially life-threatening pregnancies (Tietze 1984).

For each death from unsafe abortion, there were many women who suffered complications. Complete statistics on the number of such complications during the 1960s are unavailable, but hospital studies found marked decreases in the number of women treated for abortion complications. For example, in municipal hospitals in New York City, for each 1,000 births there were 234 admissions for incomplete spontaneous and induced abortions in 1969 and 130 such admissions in 1971 after the abortion restrictions were repealed. At least five studies in other groups of hospitals found similar decreases.

Because legalisation made abortion more accessible to the youngest and oldest women of childbearing age and those in poor health, one effect was to reduce the rate of infant mortality and premature birth. A study by economists associated with the National Bureau of Economic Research found that the increase in the abortion rate was the most important factor in explaining the reduction in neonatal mortality between 1964 and 1977. The abortion rate dominated other public policies, including Medicaid, subsidised family planning services, and maternal and infant care projects, in explaining the mortality decline among both white and black women (Joyce 1987). Other economists found that abortion also reduced the rate of low birthweight and preterm births (Grossman and Jacobowitz 1981).

## Unsafe abortion in Great Britain

Abortion was legal in the early months of pregnancy until 1803. Four years after, an advertisement in *Bells Court and Fashionable Magazine* (September 1807) claimed:

> Lost happiness regained – any lady of respectability involved in distress from any expectation of inevitable dishonour, may obtain consolation and security and a real friend in the hour of anxiety and peril by addressing a line (post paid) to Mrs Grimston no 18 Broad Street, Golden Square, when a private interview with the advertiser will be appointed. Ladies thus situated may depend on the strictest secrecy and motherly attention, combined with every comfort so necessary on these occasions for the restoration of that serenity of mind generally attendant on the cultivated life (*Lancet* 21 May 1932).

The herb, savin, was mentioned in 1837 as being the most commonly used abortifacient although a Professor Thompson felt it occurred more amongst the middling and poorer classes who would find it difficult to conceal an unwanted pregnancy: 'Should pregnancy in the unmarried female of rank take place, the disgrace can be more easily concealed.' Other doctors argued that abortion was common. By 1841 at least there were illegal operators. One doctor wrote in 1844 that he had attended three women who had aborted themselves with herbs in the previous three months. He said it was not surprising that a woman wished to avoid a 'lifetime in the dreaded union house'. By the 1850s, in addition to herbs there was also evidence of abortionists. The *Lancet* complained that 'as a trade it is carried out to a frightful extent'. (21 May 1853). A few months later it returned to the subject and complained that handbills were being addressed to female domestics telling them how to get abortions (30 July). In 1861 the *Lancet* published another editorial on the subject stating that abortion had become a money-making activity (23 March).

In 1868 there was a major investigation into abortion as a feature of baby farming by the *British Medical Journal (BMJ)*. Baby farming was the practice by which women would pay a person a sum of around £5 to adopt their children and raise them in baby farms. The investigator presented himself as representing someone who was pregnant. He was told by the proprietress that if the lady were not too far gone the affair could be handled for a sum of money with perfect safety. She continued to say that it was 'hard that people could not have a little enjoyment without being put to such inconvenience afterwards' (8 February 1868). Another place charged 50 guineas for the doctor and 20 for the proprietor and said that the woman could remain veiled if she wished. This woman said she had been in the business since 1851 and that she was never short of clients, some of whom had gone back six or seven times. The *BMJ* quoted her: 'I am a jokelar [jocular] person, I am; and I says funny things and cheers them up. She needn't mind, and mustn't fret, and I'll see her alright. I'm the old original I am, and have hundreds.' In all, the investigators visited seven establishments and six of them were willing to provide abortions.

The *BMJ* attacked ladies having abortions in part because they were setting a bad example to their maids. Under the general title of 'baby farming' the BMJ attacked other practices of the time. One was infanticide whereby the baby farmers would neglect a child until it died. Another was a curious practice in which a woman who wanted a baby would adopt one but pretend to her husband it was his. She would dress without stays to look big and when a child was found she would feign labour; the 'midwife' would buy bullock's blood from the butcher to make a mess, and the husband would be presented with a baby. The report was very revealing of Victorian sexual practices for the BMJ expressed no surprise at all that the husband could be so deceived but just complained about the transgression of the laws of primogeniture (8 February 1868).

Apart from illegal abortions there were also legal ones performed by some doctors. One doctor carried out an abortion on a woman who thought that a pregnancy might interfere with an important journey (*BMJ* 1 January 1881). Three years later the *Lancet* said there should be the strongest evidence before a doctor was brought to account for carrying out an abortion: 'the presumption was that it was done in the legal exercise of his calling' (29 March 1884).

In 1893 a women died of lead poisoning and by the early twentieth century in many areas of the country women of childbearing age presenting at hospital were routinely examined for a blue line on their gums which was indicative of lead poisoning. In an earlier book one of us called the period 1896–1914 'the abortion age' and suggested that during this time there were more actual or attempted abortions than at any time in British history (Francome 1986: 19). The evidence comes from a variety of sources. There were letters on the subject in the *BMJ* in 1898 and there was also the trial of the three Chrimes brothers. They had been advertising and in the space of two years 12,000 women replied. The brothers wrote to them under the guise of a public official saying that he was in possession of evidence that they had committed the awful crime of preventing the birth of a child and that arrest would follow unless two guineas costs were received. The blackmail was discovered and the police reported they had intercepted £800 in a few days. The brothers were sentenced to long periods in prison. The *Lancet* felt the case would end the trade but on 25 February 1899 it reported over 100 newspapers 'in which occur the advertisements of persons of whose pretensions to procure abortion there can be no doubt'. It began an aggressive campaign of 'naming and shaming' the newspapers and nearly 200 local newspapers were reported.

In many ways the best information on abortion at the beginning of the twentieth century was in the book *Report on the English Birth Rate* by Ethel Elderton (1914) based on the north of England. The evidence was concerned with the decline in the birth rate, which she felt was reducing pressure on population which 'carried the English population as the great colonising force into every quarter of the globe'. She blamed the 1877 Bradlaugh–Besant trial which, she argued, legitimised birth control and felt might be later seen as causing 'the death knell of the British Empire'. Yet her report did not show much evidence of contraception but rather that women were using abortion in a desperate attempt to control their fertility. In Bradford, for example, the birth rate had almost halved from 25 per 100 married women aged 15–55 in 1851 to 14 in 1901. Her correspondent commented: 'There is a good deal of abortion practised in this district and for every case that comes to notice there are hundreds that do not.' Elderton argued that Leeds was a great centre for fertility control and that many Leeds suppliers advertised the sale of abortifacients and the distribution of birth control information. Her fullest analysis was in the city of York where she had three correspondents. The reports were that some women obtained pills from their doctors while others took Widow Welch's female pills, colocynth, steel pills and a common remedy of gin and gunpowder. Evidence was also obtained from women. One whose husband was on poor wages and often ill said:

> Six out of ten working women take something, if it is only paltry stuff ... one tells another. There's no hawking here; its all done in secrecy ... sometimes they can take a druggist shop and it does no good ... the child comes out just the same but it's puny and half starved ... I knew a child nine months only weighed about four pounds; they kept it alive for a twelve month then it died. The mother died too ... she had been taking all sorts, and she went into rapid consumption ... Our folk go on taking what weaken them, and they can't make up for it like the rich. One woman said to me 'I'd rather swallow the druggist shop and the man in't than have another kid' (Elderton 1914: 136).

Two other working women 'of most respectable type', estimated that at least seven but probably eight out of ten working women took drugs. 'They'll rise money for that, it they rise it for nothing else ... I think nearly all of them have a try ... and there's many that half poison themselves.' Elderton suggested that while her best evidence was for York she had no doubt that it was representative of a wide range of towns. She said that in Birkenhead women asked doctors about contraception and abortion:

> Women will frankly state how they avoid pregnancy and recount how they have tried everything to bring an undesired pregnancy to a premature end. Bitter apples, lead plaster, nutmegs, etc have been taken in so many cases with acute symptoms; a few cases have been reported of attempts to introduce knitting needles into the uterus in order to produce abortion. Advertised pills are much tried (Elderton 1914: 80).

She reported the only place the birth rate had not fallen was Liverpool, which she put down to Irish immigration. Elderton's work was given extensive coverage in the *BMJ* (26 December 1914) and the *Malthusian* (January 1915). It is probable that her work was the basis of the *Malthusian*'s estimate that 100,000 working women took abortifacient pills (May 1914). The *Malthusian* also attacked the 'conspiracy of silence' which kept poor women in ignorance of harmless contraceptive devices and led them to take dangerous drugs (January 1915). Similar evidence was given to the Birth Rate Commission and one proposed that about one in four women procured abortions (1917: 2798–0).

One of the reasons for the high abortion rate was that contraception had not permeated to the working class. The socialists in Britain (but not in the USA) were opposed to it. The Malthusians said that the way to reduce poverty was to encourage people to have only as many children as they could afford. The socialists felt that there should be a change in the social order to achieve this aim (Francome 1984a).

A second reason for the high number of unwanted pregnancies was the mistiming of the safe period. It led to Ethel Elderton commenting primly: 'Most women in the country districts know that a human is more likely to be impregnated at a period around the time of menstruation and a great many avoid this time when sober' (Francome 1986: 22). This kind of knowledge was a recipe for disaster.

After the First World War, Marie Stopes and colleagues began a new approach to contraception and began promoting it as a woman's choice and not as a means to eliminate poverty. It led to a great increase in birth control use amongst the working class which had, until then, been lagging behind. In the period 1920–1924 three in five of the wives of skilled manual workers were using birth control, 4% higher than the usage of the wives of non-manual workers (Francome 1986: 23). The effect of increasing contraceptive use on the demand for abortion can be complicated. At first, expectations of control may rise faster than birth control use, so both birth control and abortion can rise together. When contraception then becomes more efficient, the demand for abortion is likely to fall. A contemporary observer concluded that this is what occurred:

> Contraceptive measures are undoubtedly one factor in lowering the incidence of the demand for abortion, and within recent years I have been rather impressed with the attitude of mind of the woman who has practised contraception and who has failed to obtain her object. Such a woman instinctively seems to feel that she has the right to demand the termination of an unwanted pregnancy (Francome 1984).

We saw that from the 1880s rich women could get abortions from doctors. This continued in the inter-war years, and the fact that a barrister's wife was given abortion on request was discussed openly at the section of obstetrics at the annual meeting of the British Medical Association. There was no attempt at secrecy but rather a discussion of grounds (*BMJ* August 1926).

For poor women there were a variety of abortifacient pills and in 1929 the Advertising Association sent a letter to all newspapers asking them to refuse such advertisements. However, these pills remained on sale until the new law was implemented in 1968. Also in 1929 was the first mention in the British medical literature of slippery elm bark, which was obtained from a tree in North America and which expanded when the bark was soaked in water. Other people used the illegal abortionist who would either use a syringe or insert an instrument of some kind. Probably the best evidence of the frequency of the different methods is the study by Parish of 1,000 abortion cases in 1930–1932. A total of 485 admitted illegal interference and in only 246 cases was Parish sure there was no intervention. Two in five used both drugs and a syringe, a quarter used only drugs, and a quarter used only a syringe. One in 25 used slippery elm bark (Parish 1935).

In some places at least the illegal abortionist was a highly respected member of the community, particularly by the women she had helped. It is not difficult to see why. In 1926 Lord Buckmaster gave the House of Lords the following case history: 'A woman was married at the age of seventeen who by the age of thirty-four had had eighteen pregnancies and eleven live children.' Buckmaster asserted that this case was not unusual. In 1930 a woman called Mrs Lee was sentenced to five years' penal servitude. She had charged up to ten shillings for an abortion and had unfortunately killed two women. Nevertheless she had the support of the local community and the newspaper reported:

> A big demonstration began when Mrs. Lee was taken away from the Shire Hall. The crowd, which consisted mainly of women, cheered when Mrs. Lee in the charge of a wardress, came out of a rear door of the Shire Hall and many crowded round he car. A sobbing woman, apparently a relative of Mrs. Lee, insisted on kissing her before she was helped into the motor which was waiting. Another woman pushed her way towards Mrs. Lee saying 'let me kiss her, I must kiss her.' From the car Mrs. Lee waved kisses to her friends and as the car left the precincts of the Shire Hall the cheering was renewed.

> There was great anger against the witnesses who caused Mrs. Lees' conviction. The cheering was changed to 'booing' when witnesses in the case were seen at the windows of the building, and shouts such as 'come out of it!' and 'Come down you dogs' were heard' (*Gloucester Journal* 14 June 1930).

In the period 1926–1935 there were 400–500 deaths each year. The number then fell away until just before the Second World War (Francome 1986: 24).

The British Medical Association (BMA) published a special report on abortion in 1936; one of the members of the committee, Aleck Bourne, carried out an abortion on a 14-year-old girl who had been raped, thus helping to establish rape as a ground for abortion. This is still part of the law in Northern Ireland (Francome 1986: 25). The BMA report led to the Birkett Committee, appointed in 1937 to investigate the prevalence of abortion. It reported that 'the law relating to abortion is freely disregarded amongst women of all types and classes' (1939: 118). It estimated there were 44,000–66,000 a year (Birkett 1939). David Glass argued that 100,000 was nearer the mark and it was his figure that was given the most publicity after the Second World War.

When the servicemen returned home there was a large increase in births but there was still demand for abortion. A useful study was that of Moya Woodside, who interviewed 44 inmates at the London women's prison at Holloway who had been convicted of illegal abortion. Many had a good safety record but others were discovered only after they had caused a death. She found the most common method of abortion was the Higginson's syringe, which 35 of them had used, usually inserting soapy water and a disinfectant. Woodside commented that money was not the primary motive but rather 'compassion and feminine solidarity' (Woodside 1963).

In post-war years the Bourne ruling had meant that Harley street doctors could be more open than hitherto; before the Abortion Act there were many legal or semi-legal abortions. An estimated 5,700 NHS abortions were carried out under what was known as the Bourne amendment. In addition, 15,000 abortions were estimated to have been performed by doctors privately (Potts et al. 1977). Further abortions were carried out in Scotland where the law was different. Dugald Baird pointed out (unpublished letter to Vera Houghton 9 March 1964) that no action could be taken against a doctor unless a complaint was made. Overall, the estimate of 100,000 abortions a year continued to be the dominant one used. In the event, after legalisation the levelling out of the figures at around this level suggests that it was about right (Francome 1977).

## Conclusion

The evidence presented here concerns Britain and the USA and shows clearly that illegal abortion was common. In neither country did significant numbers of people practise abstinence to avoid unwanted pregnancy. We have not investigated the situation in other countries to the same extent, but we have noted some important indicators. We know that in 1904 eight Italian midwives were convicted of 'abortion mongering' and that in Paris, France there were an estimated 50,000 abortions a year in 1913 – many of these for English abortion tourists (Francome 1984a: 34). We also know that in Sweden, despite a slight liberalisation of the law in 1921, there were about 60 abortion-related deaths each year in the early 1930s out of a population of 6 million (Francome 1984a: 73). There is little doubt that, just as abortions are now carried out worldwide, either safely or unsafely, this was also the case in the past. We cannot eliminate abortion and so the issue must be to develop policies which aim to give women the information and choices to reduce the necessity for terminations.

# THE POSITIVE CONSEQUENCES OF LEGALISING ABORTION

## Marcel Vekemans

*SOUTH AFRICAN INFORMATION SHOWS THAT
LIBERALISING THE ABORTION LAW IN 1997
RESULTED IN A DECREASE IN ABORTION MORTALITY
OF MORE THAN 90% BETWEEN 1996 AND 2000.*

**De Jonge et al. 1999**

With a legal abortion there is little risk to the woman's health. The related mortality is less than one in 100,000 procedures and there are few complications. If the abortion is performed before 12 weeks, the associated mortality and morbidity are much lower than those of a full-term delivery (Faúndes and Barzelatto 2006).

While there are few major health concerns related to safe abortion, there can be ethical problems adduced such as the perceived necessity to protect new human life. In reality, the issue is not so much about protecting life but about controlling female reproductive function and sexuality. Indeed, most so-called 'pro-lifers' do not actively defend human life by opposing the death penalty, war, or environmental degradation, although the Roman Catholic Church does oppose the death penalty (Francome 1978). Nor do they support contraception to prevent unwanted pregnancies, or universal access to health care. Nor do they fight neonatal death which, worldwide, accounts for four million mostly preventable deaths yearly; nor diseases that kill infants, such as malaria.

For many people restricting access to abortion is rooted in traditional patriarchal systems kept alive by laws, governments, judicial systems and religions. However, more and more leaders, governments and members of the general public understand that the death toll and the morbidity related to unsafe abortion is not acceptable and that imposed childbearing is a serious denial of a woman's right to bodily autonomy.

Thus, many organisations and individuals actively promote the right for all women to access safe abortion, and many publications address the issue. But while a great part of the literature analyses the negative consequences of restricted access to safe abortion, few concentrate on the many positive consequences of liberalising access to safe abortion. This chapter describes these positive consequences:

### Safe abortion promotes health

It improves quality of life and benefits women and families. For some women, an abortion is the first occasion they start using modern contraception. Pre- and post-abortion care includes (and must include) contraceptive counselling. During this consultation women who have experienced contraceptive failure will be reminded of its benefits and will update their knowledge. Their partners, if present, will also benefit. A method will be chosen and therefore legal abortion results in an increase in contraceptive use, which in turn results in declining abortion rates (Boonstra et al. 2006). All contraceptive methods can be used after an abortion. Repeat abortions will thus be avoided, although we know that a minority of women will need them because contraceptive methods are not perfect, nor, of course, are the users. It has been shown that women asking for repeat abortions are much more often in difficult social conditions, decreasing their autonomy and capacity for decision making. For some, repeat abortion is a distress signal. For delaying or ending childbearing, and for avoiding unwanted pregnancy, imposed pregnancy or unwanted children, abortion is a back-up method. Millions of women all over the world rely on it to manage their fertility, and so abortion should be regarded as a necessary reproductive health service. Even in countries such as the Netherlands with widespread information, good access to contraceptive services, and low abortion rates, access to safe abortion is a requisite for the female population's healthy reproductive and sexual life (Berer 2000).

Sometimes, unwanted pregnancies can be related to circumstances totally out of a woman's control. This could be, for example, the non-existence of access to comprehensive sexual information and education. Some women are the victim of abstinence-only education. Pregnancy can also be the consequence of coercive sex, including incest and rape (sometimes as a weapon of war). Many women are unable to make decisions about sex and contraceptive use in places where gender inequality persists (Berer 2000). In all such circumstances, access to safe abortion permits a secondary prevention of unfortunate or even disastrous personal or social outcomes.

Some abortions are motivated by health reasons either of the pregnant woman or of the fetus. These reasons include fetal malformations or impairment, the risk of seriously worsening of a disease the pregnant woman suffers from (e.g. cancer or some eye diseases), or when the continuation of pregnancy is contraindicated because the woman has been exposed to drugs, products or irradiations that could cause fetal malformations. In such circumstances, a woman can be confronted with a difficult choice. The possibility of accessing safe abortion gives the woman, or the couple, the opportunity to make a dignified and free choice, and to take personal responsibility.

### Legal abortion can result in a decrease in the number of abortions

There is no systematic relation between the legalisation of abortion and the number performed. With legalisation there is an initial effect of an increase in recorded numbers as legal abortions replace hidden illegal ones. There is probably also an increase in the number of abortions actually occurring as safe services become available. But over the longer term the experience of the developed world and the more limited information from developing countries shows that abortion rates often decline (Henshaw et al. 1999).

Five countries in Western Europe (Belgium, Germany, the Netherlands, Spain and Switzerland) have very low abortion rates (less than ten per thousand women of reproductive age) and all have very liberal abortion laws. They also have sex education and high use of contraception. There is, in fact, no correlation between legality and abortion rates, because so many factors influence the figures. These include the number of children wanted or accepted, the level of contraceptive use, and the quality of the studies and of the statistics.

### Abortion improves the quality of life

When a woman becomes pregnant, and the circumstances make it difficult or almost impossible to continue the pregnancy, or to look after a child, accessing safe abortion can be essential to ensure the woman a healthy, decent future life. Many situations illustrate this point: adolescents will not be obliged to leave school; students will be able to complete their studies; couples, women or families will not be plunged into poverty; heavily impaired fetuses will be saved from very difficult lives. Accessing safe abortion will increase the probability of continuing productive lives for women, couples and families (Bailey et al. 2001). Maintaining one's life prospects helps women avoid the adverse psychological effects that occur amongst women denied abortion (Dagg 1991; Faúndes and Barzelatto 2006). When abortion is legal, partners can have an honest dialogue about a problem pregnancy and consider their options. In the case of young adolescents we can avoid children having children. These adolescents can then have their children later in life when they are far better able to care for them. Those women suffering from rape or incest will not be forced to either have an unsafe abortion or to bring a child into a very difficult social situation. In the USA, 1% of abortions occur after rape and 0.5% after incest (Finer et al. 2005). In countries such as South Africa where violence on women is even more prevalent, the corresponding figures are much higher (Abrahams 2004).

### Every child a wanted child

When abortion becomes legal, a decline in adoptions occurs. This supports the conclusions that abortion legalisation leads to a reduction in the number of unwanted children (Bitler and Zavodny 2002).

### Legal abortion can help reach demographic objectives

In the context of national policies to stabilise population, promoting the use of effective means of contraception – instead of using abortion – is the best means to reach a desired policy goal. At the same time, while supporting contraception, governments should also ensure access to legal, voluntary and safe abortion. In countries where fertility was historically at high levels, access to abortion has been demonstrated by demographers to be a significant contributor to declining fertility and slower population growth (Bongaarts 1997). The demographic changes have in turn been shown to facilitate economic growth, poverty reduction and sustainable development (Bongaarts 1997). In summary, women (and partners) who can regulate their fertility can take advantage of opportunities for education, employment and general empowerment in life, and maintain their productivity and their contributions to society.

### Health care providers will improve attitudes and practices

Where abortion is legal, physicians and paramedics can provide abortion services without fearing judicial consequences. This results in far more positive attitudes among health care workers towards induced abortion, and improves their interactions with clients and patients. There can be confidence between provider and client. Conscientious objection can be addressed as long as the objectors respect the women's freedom by referring them to colleagues who will provide the treatment they need. Only if the society has a liberal attitude towards abortion will the providers have a respectful attitude to women with unwanted pregnancies.

Where abortion is illegal, there may be discrimination against women presenting for abortion as well as mistreatment and inadequate care during post-abortion visits. It has been shown that the attitude of providers is influenced by the criminalisation of induced abortion (Faúndes and Barzelatto 2006; Langer et al. 1999). Some women even prefer the privacy of clandestine abortions to the embarrassment and inconvenience associated with the use of public health services.

The attitude of some providers is open to criticism. There have been many cases of people who publicly censure abortion but privately perform them, sometimes at a huge price. We have all heard about physicians refusing abortions in the public hospital in the morning but performing them in their private practice in the afternoon. This negative image of doctors vanishes where abortion is legalised.

### There are more understanding attitudes in the public

Where abortion is illegal there is often a dichotomy between a public condemnation and a private acceptance when a termination is for oneself, one's daughter, one's family member, one's friend, one's spouse or one's girlfriend. Many safe abortion practitioners have been faced with abortion demands from persons who are close relatives of anti-choice politicians, leaders or even religious figures. When abortion becomes legal, a progressive shift to a more positive attitude occurs. Indeed, the legalisation of abortion avoids acute conflicts between pro-choice and anti-choice people, because the recourse to the intervention becomes a private matter between a woman or a couple and the health care providers. The existence of clinics with integrated abortion and reproductive health services, as compared with clinics specialising only in abortion, helps to increase discretion around abortion, and so reduces any stigmatisation. Progressively, public opinion understands the advantages that result from access to safe abortion. Fewer conflicts with prevailing social norms arise. In most Western European countries with liberal abortion laws the abortion debate has cooled off, and anti-choice movements are less vocal or non-existent.

Police officers confronted with rape, incest or gender violence can take a positive approach in the case of an unwanted pregnancy and discuss emergency contraception and legal abortion.

## Access to safe abortion can help to reach the Millennium Development Goals

At the United Nations Millennium Summit, in 2000, 191 countries agreed on the need to reduce poverty and inequality worldwide. An important goal is to improve maternal health (Goal 5). This goal is rightly associated with abortion, because, as we have seen, 13% of maternal deaths are due to the complications of unsafe abortion. These deaths are almost totally preventable by allowing and ensuring access to safe abortion.

Abortion is in fact linked to numerous Millennium Development Goals. Goal 1 aims at eradicating extreme poverty and hunger and safe abortion can be used to improve the economic survival of a family or an individual. Clearly, the determinants of a woman's socio-economic status are varied, but women who can regulate their fertility, including accessing safe abortion, can take advantage of opportunities for education, employment and political empowerment, and have a greater ability to achieve and maintain overall health and wellbeing and be better able to contribute to society (Crane and Hord 2006). Goal 3 aims to promote gender equality and empower women. This relates evidently to the right of a woman to make decisions for herself. This will be developed more in detail below. Goal 4 aims to reduce child mortality. If a woman dies after an unsafe abortion, the probability that her existing children will die is increased. Goal 6 aims at combating HIV/AIDS, malaria and other diseases. While the links here with abortion are less evident, they do exist. Women living with HIV who become pregnant have had a varied response. Sometimes they have been allowed to abort; others have been forbidden to use their situation as grounds for legal abortion. In addition, the costs of treating diseases in general and HIV in particular can prevent a family from having (more) children. Goal 8 aims at developing a Global Partnership for Development. One could say that there is a huge need for global partnership to make progress in ensuring universal access to safe legal abortion.

Overall, the promotion of safe legal abortion will aid countries in contributing to the Millennium objectives.

## Access to safe abortion improves human rights and gender equality

The ability to decide on a personal matter as important as whether or not to bear a child is essential to a woman's human rights and has direct implications on the achievement of gender equality (Crane and Hord 2006). While nature places special burdens on women, laws should not place additional ones. Access to safe and legal abortion is a woman's human right. International legal support for a woman's right to safe and legal abortion can be found in numerous international treaties. A list of such treaties is available online (CRR 2004).

The issue of accessing safe and legal abortion is connected to many aspects of human rights: the right to health and reproductive health; the right to decide the number and spacing of children; the right to marry and to found a family; the right to life, liberty and security; the right to be free from gender discrimination and sexual assault; the right to be free from cruel, inhumane or degrading treatment or punishment; the right to privacy; and the right to enjoy scientific progress (CRR 2004).

In addition there is the right to information. Sex education, for both sexes, should include discussing the issue of abortion. However, only if safe abortion is accessible can this education be complete. Where safe abortion is not accessible, the issue is avoided or addressed only in a stigmatising way, which does not help to address the problem. Owing to religious doctrine or concern with freer sexuality many countries opposed to abortion also oppose the use of contraception, which would reduce its incidence. Furthermore many countries oppose safe abortion but also oppose financial support for pregnant women which might enable them to continue the pregnancy.

Laws that ban abortion prevent a woman from exercising her right to access a procedure that may be necessary for her enjoying her right to health, her right to regulate her fertility, her right to decide for herself. Denying access to safe legal abortion restricts women to a subordinate position in their family and community. Where abortion is illegal, women are exposed to health risks not experienced by men, and cannot make responsible decisions about their lives (CRR 2004).

### Legal abortion helps develop the capacity to make choices

The decision as to whether or not to continue with a pregnancy should rest with the woman. She should be able to ask for information on the procedures. Furthermore, counselling should be available if she needs help in making her decision. These rights to information and assistance are fundamental but can only be met in a context of liberal access to safe abortion, the woman being empowered and able to control her own fate. Protecting a woman's right, as a full moral agent, to decide in conscience to continue or terminate her pregnancy is simply, but importantly, showing respect for women. President Bachelet from Chile put it rightly, at the UN General Assembly in 2006: 'The State only gives the option. The persons decide by their own values, by their own beliefs. We don't impose anything on anyone.'

### Abortion rights can reduce inequality

If abortion is legal the 'principle of justice' means there should be no discrimination between patients. There should be equal access to safe services for rich and poor, rural and urban, and all categories of people with special problems or needs. Indeed, access to safe abortion removes the injustice of the unpalatable 'safe, costly abortion available to women of means, but unavailable to the poor' (Bhuiya et al. 2001). A study in Egypt illustrates this fact. It was found that unsafe abortion cost less than one dollar while a safe illegal abortion cost 2.5 times the average per capita monthly income (Lane et al. 1998). Legalising abortion aids respect for positive legal principles. Decriminalising abortion respects an elementary principle of justice: equality. Everyone can access the service. In countries where access to abortion is restricted, the wealthy can obtain it locally or by travelling to a neighbouring country, while the poor cannot.

### Legal abortion spares many people the cruelty of jail

We have seen that women and providers have been severely punished for breaking abortion laws. Legalisation suppresses this cruelty and saves the related costs for the victims as well as for the penal establishment. The most effective way to reduce the human, social and economic costs of abortion is to abolish the laws that penalise it (Faúndes and Barzelatto 2006).

### Legalised abortion shows that respect for minority rights prevails

We discussed in the Introduction that it is perfectly possible for a religious or political leader to take the view that while in their own lives they may be opposed to abortion, nevertheless there should still be provision for those who do not share their point of view. In Catholic countries, the decriminalisation of abortion is proof of a healthy separation between Church and State, and a proof also that non-Catholic minorities can live according to their own value system. In addition, Catholics themselves will be able to decide according to their conscience rather than to rigid Church rules. Church teaching supports the right of Catholics to disagree with its teachings and to follow their own conscience. The catechism states that 'In all he says and does, man [*sic*] is obliged to follow faithfully what he knows to be just and right.' From this there is a case for saying that a Catholic woman who follows her conscience and decides that having an abortion is in the best interest of her and the rest of her family commits no sin. This is true even though the objective judgement of the Church that abortion is a sin remains intact. This is because a central tenet of Roman Catholic faith – one's conscience, honestly formed – supersedes other influences (Kissling 2006).

A liberal abortion law does not oblige anybody to abort, but shows respect for the minority of women who choose this option. The respect of minorities is one of the main characteristics of democracy.

### Countries with liberal abortion laws comply with conventions

Organisations like the United Nations, the Council of Europe and the European Union have made calls to action (IPPF 2006). Countries which have signed up to these should respect their commitments. An important feature is that countries should ensure access to abortion to the fullest extent of what their law permits. This depends on the government and on the judiciary, but also strongly on the attitude of the health care providers, especially the physicians, and of their professional associations (Rahman et al. 1998).

### The legalisation of abortion can be a break from a colonial past

Many developing countries had laws based on the laws of their occupying powers. These were normally restrictive laws introduced by countries which have almost universally changed their own laws and allowed access to legal abortion.

### Legalising abortion allows a shifting energy to reducing the number

Instead of spending resources fighting anti-choice organisations, more effort is available to empower women in their sexual activity, to educate both sexes and to provide information about contraceptive methods (Faúndes and Barzelatto 2006).

### Legal abortion allows quality research on abortion and related issues

Illegal abortion is extremely difficult to investigate, as only the most dangerous consequences can be documented through clinical studies. Furthermore, abortion can be part of the medical curriculum and doctors become more skilled in performance (Faúndes and Barzelatto 2006). At the moment accurate statistics about abortion are scarce. One of the most complete analyses of the global incidence of abortion identified only 28 countries, of which 20 are in Europe, with data 'believed to be complete' (Henshaw et al. 1999).

## Legal abortion results in a decrease in second trimester abortions, which entail more complications

This has been shown in the USA after the 1973 legalisation of abortion (Boonstra et al. 2006). Yet there is still a need for second trimester services to be available on health grounds. At one hospital the frequency of abortion complications decreased dramatically after legalisation, but when the hospital stopped providing second-trimester abortion the rate of complications increased markedly. This and similar evidence demonstrates how important it is to ensure access to safe abortion also in the second trimester of pregnancy (De Jonge et al. 1999; Dickson-Tetteh and Rees 1999; Rees et al. 1997).

## Liberal abortion reduces maternal mortality

I discussed this briefly under the Millennium Goals (Berer 2004; Susser 1992). Unsafe abortion leads to medical complications with the main consequences being mortality, physical complications (haemorrhage, anaemia, transfusion – sometimes with HIV contamination – infection, pelvic inflammatory disease, peritonitis, septicaemia, traumatic and chemical lesions, toxic reactions, shock; removal of tubes, ovaries, uterus; tubal obstruction, ectopic pregnancy, sterility, chronic pelvic pain and interferences with sexual intercourse due to pain and libido decrease). These problems can have severe psychological and major negative social consequences such as repudiation, divorce, violence or marginalisation (Faúndes and Barzelatto 2006; Ladipo 1989; Liskin 1992).

Evidence from Romania has been given; similarly South African information shows that liberalising the abortion law in 1997 resulted in a decrease in abortion mortality of more than 90% between 1996 and 2000 (De Jonge et al. 1999; Dickson-Tetteh and Rees 1999; Jewkes et al. 2005; Rees et al. 1997). At the same time, more studies from South Africa have shown that while legalisation of abortion immediately decreased morbidity, there is a need to ensure the suppression of additional covert induced abortion activity, to train providers (physicians and midwives) extensively, and to introduce modern techniques such as vacuum aspiration, proper use of antibiotics, pain relief techniques and less use of general anaesthesia (Jewkes et al. 2005). In 1995, in Guyana, the number of hospital admissions for complications from unsafe abortion decreased by 41% during the six months after the legalisation of post-abortion care (Nunes and Delph 1997).

In England and Wales, there were around 80 deaths related to induced abortion during the three years before the liberalisation of abortion, and no deaths during the three years after (Stephenson et al. 1992). In New York, there was a 50% drop in the number of abortion-related deaths in the two years after the liberalisation of the law (Tietze al. 1972), and in the USA as a whole a dramatic decrease in abortion-related deaths occurred after the 1973 liberalisation of abortion (Cates et al. 2003). Research in more than 160 countries has shown that where legislation allows abortion in a broad range of cases (as compared with countries with restrictive legislation), there is a lower incidence of unsafe abortion (Berer 2004).

On average, in all developing regions (excluding China), the yearly rate of hospital admissions resulting from unsafe abortion is 5.7 per thousand women aged 15–44. There are regional variations, but not very large: in eastern and southern Africa the corresponding figure is 10; in western Africa 6; in northern Africa 12; in south-central Asia 4; in south-east Asia 3; in western Asia 8; in Latin America 8; in the Caribbean 3. Translated in absolute figures, there are 1,700,000 hospitalisations in Africa, 2,300,000 in Asia (without China), 2,300,000 in Latin America, and 1,000,000 in the Caribbean. A country such as Brazil has to provide care for 250,000 women admitted to hospital each year because of abortion complications (Singh 2006). The above figures are very rough, of course, given the clandestine nature of unsafe abortion. Also, some statistics do not distinguish between the consequences of spontaneous and induced abortion. In addition to these depressing figures, it has been shown that worldwide 15–25% of all women undergoing unsafe abortions have complications but do not obtain the necessary treatment (Guttmacher Institute 1999).

Where abortion is illegal, the use of safer self-inducing abortion methods, such as taking (correctly) misoprostol, and access to emergency primary health care 24 hours a day, in addition to the provision of quality post-abortion care, using aspiration and antibiotics, decreases the impact of complications in terms of costs and suffering (Singh 2006). Misoprostol must however be used cautiously. When administered clinically, it is highly effective (Carbonell et al. 1997), but when self-administered, and either not monitored or monitored less closely, it is less effective (Blanchard et al. 2000; Koopersmith and Mishell 1996) and can be dangerous in case of overdosage or even cause death (Henriques et al. 2007).

Estimates have been made of the disability burden of unsafe abortion using an indicator called DALYs (Disability-Adjusted Life Years), which integrates the loss of productive life resulting from both death and illness. Unsafe abortion is responsible for the loss of about 5 million years of productive life, i.e. 14% of all DALYs lost from pregnancy-related conditions. This burden has probably been greatly underestimated, as many women who have complications do not seek or receive medical care, and as the long-term impact of unsafe abortion on women's health, through such conditions as infertility, are difficult to quantify (Abou-Zhar and Vaughan 2000; Singh 2006; Singh et al. 2003; WHO 2002).

Fortunately, long-term campaigns by women's health advocates have led to increased willingness of hospitals and health care providers to treat incomplete abortions and to a lessening in women's fears of seeking care (Singh 2006). But unsafe abortion in the second trimester remains a source of serious complications since it still accounts for many of the hospital admissions (Singh 2006). The necessity for the provision of adequate post-abortion care was foreseen in the 1994 International Conference on Population and Development (ICPD) Cairo proceedings: 'In all cases women should have access to quality services for the management of complications arising from abortion' (UN 1995). In countries with restrictive laws an intermediary step to decrease the morbidity and mortality related to unsafe abortion is to ensure that post-abortion care can be provided easily and safely, without any denunciation to police or judiciary by medical, administrative or other staff in the health care facility. And women who have had an abortion should not be prosecuted. It would be unethical for the medical profession not to respect strict confidentiality in relation to post-abortion care.

### Access to safe abortion has additional health benefits

Access to safe abortion helps sick women to avoid having children (e.g. women who are HIV positive or suffer from AIDS) (Vekemans and da Silva 2005), or risking dangerous pregnancy-related illnesses (such as eclampsia, or post-partum psychosis). It avoids the use of those traumatising and dangerous traditional abortion-inducing methods (e.g. ingestion of poisonous substances, trauma to the abdomen, insertion of objects into the uterus).

Post-abortion care, which includes the treatment of complications arising from spontaneous abortion (miscarriage), can be provided without hesitation, using modern technology, in the same way as that used for the treatment of complications after induced abortion. Even the treatment of ectopic pregnancy will be improved: providers are no longer fearful of breaking the law in performing aspiration or curettage in pregnant women presenting with medical complications.

### Liberal abortion has economic advantages

It reduces the cost of health care. By providing safe abortion services, public health systems will save the high costs of treating complications of unsafe abortion in already over-burdened hospital facilities. This will free resources to address other critical health needs of the low-income populations they serve. Costs to provide treatment for unsafe or incomplete abortion can run in the order of ten times as high as providing women with early elective abortion services at a primary care level in their community (H Johnston unpublished).

An illustrative study from Tanzania estimated that the cost per day of providing post-abortion care was more than seven times the annual amount allocated by the Ministry of Health for per capita health expenses (Mpangile et al. 1993). Shifting resources that could be saved by legalising abortion to other essential preventative measures and obstetric care for poor women could go a long way toward improving their reproductive health status and wellbeing (Konje et al. 1992). In the capital city of Burkina Faso, Ouagadougou, the city's hospitals treated in 2004 an estimated 1,100 abortion complications (Rossier et al. 2004). In Maputo, Mozambique, the treatment of a patient with abortion complications costs nine times more than a safe abortion in the same hospital and five times the cost of a normal delivery (Faúndes and Barzelatto 2006). More in-depth analysis of the economic and social costs of unsafe abortion to women and to the health system could still be conducted (Singh 2006). In addition to the savings made in the health care system through the decriminalisation of abortion, there are savings in the social costs: decreases in individual and familial poverty, and in the number of dysfunctional families. Participation of the concerned individuals in economic productivity will improve. Safe abortion permits women to keep a job that would be compromised by the arrival of an unwanted child.

### Abortion care can be part of improving all care

While legal abortion is in principle safe there are some countries where quality of care is not of the highest standard. On the other hand, safe abortions can be obtained (often at high cost) in countries where abortion is restricted. Thus, the use of the terms 'unsafe' and 'safe' abortions must be kept distinct from 'legal' and 'illegal' abortions (Faúndes and Barzelatto 2006). We have seen that in some countries such as Vietnam, where abortion is legal, the access to safe abortion can still be limited.

## Conclusion

Despite the evidence of widespread unsafe abortion and the history of illegal abortion, anti-choice people still believe that legal prohibition would reduce the number of abortions and that keeping an unwanted child or giving a child up for adoption is better than abortion. It is true that sometimes continuing the pregnancy will result in a happy ending, but the evidence is that statistically there are more troubled children, resulting in ill-adapted adults, after unwanted pregnancies (Dagg 1991; Faúndes and Barzelatto

2006; Matejcek et al. 1985).

By allowing a woman to weigh the moral considerations relevant to the decision to continue or terminate her pregnancy, liberal abortion laws effectively give her full citizenship. Only when women have the right of reproductive choice and the ability to control their own fertility can they participate equally in their nation's social, political and economic life (Borgmann and Weiss 2003).

Positive results from liberalising abortion laws or decriminalising abortion can be used by advocates, health care providers and policymakers to increase awareness of the public health burden of unsafe abortion and to build political commitment to reduce it. Unsafe abortion is almost entirely preventable, and the means of preventing it are known. We have seen that prevention not only decreases the rates of unsafe abortions, but can also reduce the number of safe abortions. We will be arguing that the elimination of unsafe abortion is a critical priority for the developing world.

Many pro-choice advocates propose to take abortion altogether out of the penal code. They take the view that there is no need for any other regulation than the rules which apply to medical acts in general. The proposal is that abortion should be provided in the same way as any other health service and, as such, monitored by professional organisations. Complete decriminalisation exists in Canada and the Capital Territory in Australia and it seems that it allows a restrained approach to the issue, with excellent results for public health. 'No abortion law' can result in earlier access (when the procedure is safest), as there is no 'waiting time' as is mandatory in many countries. There could be problems in that the right to access safe abortion is not guaranteed if many or most practitioners and hospitals decide not to perform them or set low time limits. However, overall it seems the benefits will outweigh the problems.

# CONCLUSIONS AND RECOMMENDATIONS

*FUNDS WILL BE CHANNELED TO RELIGIOUS GROUPS ADVOCATING ABSTINENCE UNTIL MARRIAGE AND REFUSING TO DISTRIBUTE CONDOMS.*

*Guardian* **2007**

In the rich countries we can distinguish four groups. In countries like Belgium, Holland, Germany and Switzerland there are good quality contraceptive and abortion services and low abortion rates. In some ways they may provide an example as to what can be achieved in other countries by a change of policy. Second, there are those countries which, while being rich, still have relatively high rates of unwanted pregnancy and abortion and clearly have the opportunity to improve access and reduce the demand for abortion. The UK is a good example in that when it introduced free contraception this excluded men. A change in policy with condoms being provided free through general practitioners as part of a men's health programme would not only reduce unwanted pregnancies but help reduce the incidence of sexually transmitted infections. A third group is the countries of Eastern Europe which have not had a tradition of contraception and, consequently, much higher abortion rates than exist elsewhere. Finally, the fourth group is the four developed countries – Ireland, Poland, Malta and the Vatican – which do not allow legal abortion and where women who do not want to continue a pregnancy have to become abortion tourists or, if poor, have local unsafe abortions.

Amongst the poor countries there are important regional groupings. We have seen that in Latin America there are poor contraceptive services and many unsafe abortions. However, there are signs of change, especially with the legalisation in Mexico City and the court decision in Colombia (see chapter 5). In Africa the great amount of poverty, ethnic and national differences, and often a strong gender divide indicates the need for a great injection of resources and improvement of health not only in the area of childbirth but throughout the population. Asia benefits from the fact that the dominant religions are more supportive of family planning, but the status of women is generally inferior and in need of improvement.

## Pro-choice is pro-life

We who are in the pro-choice movement are pro-life. The provision of safe legal abortion will save the lives of many thousands of mothers and enable them to care more adequately for their families. At the time a legal abortion is to be performed there is a great opportunity for educating women in the methods of modern contraception and wider health issues; this can help to reduce the number of deaths of children in infancy or in childhood. We are also in favour of women being able to use such procedures as artificial insemination by donor or in vitro fertilisation to enable childless women to have a family. We saw in the Introduction that decisions inspired by the Catholic Church in Poland have led to the closing of an in vitro fertilisation facility in Warsaw.

There are those who believe that it is possible to persuade young people to be sexually abstinent until they have finished their education and are married. If this were achievable there would be no need for abortion amongst single people. The few women who broke the norms could either keep the baby or give it up for adoption to a family who would give it good quality care. There would also be no need for abortion amongst the married for families would accept children as they came. The evidence of this book shows that there is not one society that in any way approaches this model.

There is also evidence that the US House of Representatives has been highly critical of US abstinence-only educational programmes. According to the Waxman Report, out of 13 curricula studied, 11 had scientific errors and distortions. Examples of errors were that a boy can impregnate a girl by touching her genitals, that 10% of women who undergo abortion become sterile, that 50% of gay male teenagers are HIV positive, that condoms fail to prevent HIV 31% of the time and result in pregnancy 13% of the time. The report suggested that youths who pledge abstinence are significantly less likely to make informed choices.

## Anti-abortion myths

The anti-abortionists have been misleading the population by promoting false propaganda or extreme viewpoints without public support. The following are just a few examples.

Anti-abortionists may say, 'A woman should not be able to have an abortion for rape.' In the words of Dr and Mrs Willke, 'Isn't it twisted logic that would kill an unborn baby for the crime of his father.' On 26 September 2006 the Pope said that 'abortion is never justifiable' (Westen 2006a). However, to force women to maintain such pregnancies against their will is extending the initial crime and causing further trauma. Furthermore, the evidence from the Congo has shown that children born of rape often have extremely difficult lives through rejection. It is true that sometimes Protestant anti-abortion leaders take the view that abortion should be allowed for rape and as we have seen the US gag rule allows abortion for this reason.

Some anti-abortionists say, 'When a woman has been raped most of the trauma has already occurred.' To quote Dr and Mrs Willke again: 'Will she be able to live comfortably with the memory that she killed her developing baby?' Experience suggests that she can. For example, in 1938, after Dr Aleck Bourne performed an abortion on a girl aged 14 who had been raped, she was ever grateful to him and 30 years afterwards sent him a letter of thanks.

Anti-abortionists may oppose state funding for family planning. For example, Robert G Marshall, legislative counsel for the so called US Coalition for Life, stated in his testimony before Congress on the extension of the Health Services Act 1977: 'We are opposed to the continued funding of the so-called family planning services and Population Research Act ... Both the IUD and one mode of action of the current pill are abortifacients.' Yet scientific studies show that the IUD works primarily by preventing fertilisation and oral contraceptives by blocking ovulation. In any case, we take the view that if poor people do not have the right to control their own fertility they are denied an essential freedom. We can agree with the US Supreme Court comments (22 January 1973):

> We recognize the right of the individual, married or single, to be free from the unwarranted governmental intrusion into matters so fundamentally affecting a person as the decision whether to bear or beget a child. That right necessarily included the right of a woman to decide whether or not to terminate a pregnancy.

Anti-abortionists may believe that the availability of birth control and abortion may lead to promiscuity. In Britain the evidence from the Brook Advisory Service, which specialises in providing services to young people, shows that over 90% of single people attending have already had intercourse.

Anti-abortionists may argue that the dissemination of knowledge of birth control will not reduce unwanted pregnancies. For example, on the fifth anniversary of the Supreme Court's decision legalising abortion, Bishop Joseph Bernadin wrote in the *New York Times* that he very much doubted whether:

more and better contraceptive information and services will make major inroads in the number of teenage pregnancies … [for] It will motivate them to precocious sexual activity but by no means the practice of contraception. In which case the 'solution' will merely have made the problem worse (Francome 1984).

Yet we have seen many countries have improved contraceptive usage and reduced the number of unwanted pregnancies. For example, in England and Wales from 1970 to 1980 the teenage birth rate fell by two-fifths as contraception and sex education improved. Only one-seventh of the decline was due to abortion (Francome 1983). In countries such as Russia and the Ukraine, contraceptive services have improved in recent years and abortion has become less common.

They say, 'Women should not be able to have an abortion or use modern methods of contraception even if there is a certainty that the resulting child would be severely handicapped.' To quote the 'Declaration on Abortion' ratified by the Pope on 28 June 1974:

> A Christian [Catholic] outlook cannot be limited to the horizon of life in this world. He [sic] knows that during the present life another one is being prepared, one of such importance that it is in this light that such judgments must be made. From this viewpoint there is no absolute misfortune here below, not even the terrible sorrow of bringing up a handicapped child. This is the contradiction proclaimed by the Lord: 'happy those who mourn: They shall be comforted'.

Some people may wish to take the risk of producing a severely disadvantaged child and to bring it up in the best way possible. They should, of course, have the total support of the community, and society should do whatever it can to provide help. But there are many people who would have great difficulty in looking after such a child and these people should have the right to choose their method of fertility control.

Anti-abortionists argue there should be no stem cell research to help the victims of Alzheimer's disease. On 26 November 2006 the Pope reiterated that he would never cease to warn of 'ethical problems of embryonic stem cell research'. US President George W Bush took a similar view, but in 2002 he was opposed by a former president's wife, Nancy Reagan. One observer called her 'one of the most revered icons of the Republican Party' and she was quoted as saying on the subject, 'A lot of time is being wasted' (Francome 2004: 94).

## Unsafe abortion is a preventable tragedy

We opened by comparing the deaths from terrorism with those from unsafe abortion. This must lead us to conclude that childbirth in general and abortion in particular are neglected problems of health care in developing countries. The moral and religious arguments around abortion have continued to obscure its importance as a serious public health problem. As a result, successful policies and strategies to reduce the unnecessary numbers of deaths resulting from unsafe abortion have not been adopted. Although following the International Conference on Population and Development (ICPD) the abortion issue has received much more attention, a lack of reliable information and data on this problem has hampered a number of activities that would have helped to ameliorate the situation.

# What can be done

## Aiding the poorer countries

We discussed governments' aid to the poor countries in the Introduction. On 30 May 2007 President Bush announced that the USA was to double spending combating HIV/AIDS in Africa and three countries elsewhere to $30 billion over five years. The reports said 'a significant part of the funds will be channeled to religious groups advocating abstinence until marriage and refusing to distribute condoms' (*Guardian* 2007). As the USA will be initiating such failed policies probably until Bush leaves office in January 2008 it behoves other countries to fill the gaps. We reported two prostitutes fighting over a used condom which they aimed to recycle, both hoping to protect their health. Such women deserve our help to safeguard themselves. The developed countries should ensure that everyone in poor countries has access to condoms either free or at low prices.

Other modern methods of contraception also need to be supported and need the rich governments to help women use the kind of contraception most convenient for them. Stan Henshaw writes:

> Few developing countries offer a complete range of contraceptive methods. Countries need female sterilization AND male sterilization AND IUD AND norplant AND pills AND patch AND ring AND condoms AND periodic abstinence because different couples have different needs. And services are needed for unmarried women and teenagers as well as others (personal communication).

## Time to change laws

The abortion debate has focused largely on the moral issues of the value of the embryo or fetus in relation to the rights of women to control their bodies and the rights of couples to limit their childbearing. Our concern here, however, is with the public health consequences of various abortion policies, and the recommendations are for policies that best promote the health of women and children.

From a public health point of view, universal access to abortion services is clearly desirable. As explained, access to legal abortion has benefits for the health of both women and children. Thus, all restrictions that have the effect of reducing the supply of abortion providers or creating barriers for women seeking services are undesirable from the point of view of public health and welfare. There is little if any health justification for restrictions on abortion services that do not apply equally to other types of health care. Public health services in developing countries should provide abortion, since low-income women have the most need for abortion services and face the greatest health risk from unwanted pregnancies. In almost all industrialised countries, government-sponsored health insurance covers abortion.

Canada provides evidence that no abortion-specific regulations are needed. The country has had no abortion law since 1988 with no ill effects on the health of women and with no excessive elevation of the abortion rate – which is lower than the rate in the USA – and no evident effect on the proportion of second-trimester abortions (Henshaw et al. 2001).

Legislation requiring special counselling for abortion, waiting periods, and parental involvement for minors serves no real purpose. If anything, women contemplating abortion need less special consideration than those planning to continue their pregnancies, since the risks and consequences of birth are greater than those of abortion. The medical profession has perceived no need for regulations specific to women seeking prenatal care, and the same reasoning should apply to women seeking to terminate their pregnancies.

As in all fields of medicine, there are some physicians who provide substandard care and who exploit certain population groups, for example, by charging excessive fees to immigrants. There is no evidence, however, that licensing requirements specific to abortion improve the quality of care, while it is inevitable that such requirements increase costs and reduce the number of providers, thereby making it more difficult for women to gain access to abortion services. Change in the restrictive laws would improve women's care.

## Education

What is clear from our analysis of the world situation is that there is no major country which has successfully persuaded its population to practise abstinence on a wide scale and for the long periods necessary in times when marriages are delayed. There are, however, a number of countries where contraceptive and health education have been such that the rates of unwanted pregnancy and abortion are greatly diminished. We have seen that in many countries there have been strong opponents of contraception. This is true for countries as disparate as India, where some recommend yoga instead, to the USA, where some teach abstinence. We would maintain that the way forward is to provide good quality information to all young people; then if some choose to be sexually abstinent they have that choice.

Even in the richer countries there are gaps in services leading to countries such as England and Wales having abortion rates twice as high as some of their continental neighbours. Hayley Blackburn of the UK's Family Planning Association writes (personal communication):

> All young people should receive high quality personal social and health education from an early age. Although the UK Government has acknowledged the role of high quality sex and relationships education in supporting efforts to reduce rates of unintended pregnancies and sexually transmitted infections, it is still not a statutory part of the curriculum at all key stages and is sadly lacking in some areas of the country. Some basic elements of human reproduction are included in the national science curriculum and there is a requirement to teach young people about HIV and sexually transmitted diseases at secondary school.

> The guidance varies between each country within the UK, which results in extremely patchy provision. Young people consistently report that the sex and relationships education they receive at school is too little, too late and too biological. To provide young people with the knowledge, skills and confidence to make informed choices about their own sexual health education must start from an early age and should achieve a balanced acquisition of:

> • **Attitudes:**
>   appreciation of difference; tolerance; openness about sex

> • **Skills:**
>   negotiation; communication; assertiveness; personal skills; managing emotions and relationships; problem-solving skills; decision-making skills

- **Knowledge:**
  puberty; the mechanics of sex, including the biological aspects; fertility and reproduction; contraception and sexually transmitted diseases; information about sexual orientation and sexuality

To ensure the quality of sexual, relationship and education provision, it is vital that the professionals responsible for its delivery are adequately trained. Some teachers do not feel comfortable teaching this material and training is required to support them to deliver it. A certification scheme for Personal, Social and Health Education, which has been introduced for teachers and school nurses, is to be welcomed. However, the FPA believes that it should be part of the core Initial Teacher Training programmes and there should be a greater focus on improving the quality and availability of post-qualification training in this area for teachers and school nurses.

There are great improvements that can be made in education in the UK and other countries are even further behind in their development.

## Time for Catholics to change

Christianity began as a religion of love. 'Love one another even as I have loved you.' The Catholic Church used to reflect this and for over a thousand years priests were able to marry and have families. The Church was tolerant of sexual behaviour as a normal part of life. However, changes occurred and the Church deviated a great deal from the early teachings of Christianity. It opposed priests and nuns having sexual relationships, criticised sex even within marriage and opposed contraception. The Catholic Church is doing some important work, for example in helping to reduce poverty, but the positive actions are being undermined by the Church's imposing standards of sexual behaviour which are unattainable for many people and which lead to social problems. One difficulty is the amount of child abuse committed by priests denied normal family life. In April 2007 the BBC announced that 400 men were abused in recent years by Catholic priests in the Dublin area of Ireland. Many more have been abused in the USA. This kind of problem will occur as long as priests are not allowed to marry and have a family.

We have seen that Catholic countries which discourage the use of modern methods of contraception tend to have high numbers of abortions. If abortion is illegal, it leads to unsafe operations. The proven way to reduce the number of abortions is to have good quality sex education, easy access to contraception and legal abortion at least in the early months of pregnancy. The Catholic Church can help facilitate this in two ways. First, it could change policy. The Church accepted abortion until 1869 and so it could revert to this position.

In recent years it has espoused the doctrine that 'life begins at conception'. This doctrine is unsustainable. Life begins before conception. Each fertile man and woman carries around with them the seeds of the future generation. With the average man carrying around 200 million live sperm only the smallest minority of these seeds will result in a live baby. So, second, if the Catholic Church is genuine about wishing to reduce the number of abortions it should support policies similar to those countries with low abortion rates. These are the countries of Europe with good contraceptive facilities which give women the right to choose in the early months of pregnancy.

Even without changing policy it could follow the example of the Catholic Priest Father Robert Drinan in Massachusetts. He was also a US Member of Congress and Dean at the Boston Law College. He took the view that it was not good for the law to make decisions as to which fetuses should be born. Rather there should be a repeal of the law:

> One way to avoid the necessity of making these choices would be for the law to withdraw its protection from *all* fetuses during the first twenty-six weeks of their existence. Under this arrangement the law would not be required to approve or disapprove the choices of parents and physicians as to who may be born or not born (Francome 1984a: 113).

This position is more or less that of most Democratic presidential hopefuls in the USA. They take the view that, while they personally may not agree with abortion, the law should not try to impose this morality. If the Catholic Church were to take this line it could maintain its position but help avoid the health problems that occur when abortion is criminalised.

As education develops, the childbearing age tends to rise and the problem of age infertility increases. Some of these women can be helped by in vitro fertilisation; others whose partners are infertile may be helped by artificial insemination by donor. So far these aids to fertility have been opposed by the Church but a change of policy towards non-intervention or approval could help many women who hitherto have not received support. A change in policy by the Church could lead to great improvement in the health of society and of family life.

The evidence shows conclusively that, worldwide, there are many 'silent' deaths of women which could be prevented through policy changes and education. As we have shown, all countries of the world have a large part to play in improving health care for pregnant women, and providing them with real choices. It is time for positive action to end the tragic and avoidable deaths of women in childbirth or abortion.

# References

Abernathy JR, Greenberg BG and Horvitz DG (1970) Estimates of induced abortion in urban North Carolina. *Demography* 7(1): 19–29.

Abou-Zhar C and Vaughan JP (2000) Assessing the burden of sexual and reproductive ill-health: questions regarding the use of disability-adjusted life years. *Bulletin of the World Health Organization* 78: 655–66.

Abrahams N (2004) Sexual violence against women in South Africa. *Sexuality in Africa* 2004 1(3):4–6. Available online at http://www.arsrc.org/downloads/sia/jan05/jan05.pdf (accessed 18 April 2007).

Acosta D (2007) Many women prefer abortions to condoms. *Inter Press Service Agency.* ipsnews.net/news.asp?idnews=33458 (accessed 24 July 2007).

Adler K (2004) New man tackles Spanish machismo. BBC News, 27 April. http://news.bbc.co.uk/1/hi/world/europe/3661117.stm (accessed 24 July 2007).

Akin A, Kocoglu GO and Akin L (2005) Study supports the introduction of early medical abortion in Turkey. *Reproductive Health Matters* 13(26): 10–19.

Al-Rabee A (2003) *Adolescent Reproductive Health in Yemen.* US Aid for International Development: New York.

Amagee LK (1999) 'Recours à l'avortement provoqué en milieu scolaire au Togo'. Paper presented at International Seminar on 'Reproductive Health in Africa', Abidjan, Cote d'Ivoire.

Amnesty International (2003) *Saudi Arabia.* Amnesty International: London.

Anderson H (1980) Abortion in Spain. *Peace News*, 25 January.

Anderson K (2001) Lives on the line. www.saidit.org/archives/May01/article/ (accessed 24 July 2007).

Arilha M and Barbosa RM (1993) Cytotec in Brazil. *Reproductive Health Matters* 1(21): 415–22.

Arthur J (1999) Legal abortion: the sign of a civilized society. www.prochoiceactionnetwork–canada.org.civilize.htm (accessed 17 July 2007).

Associated Press (2005) Chinese to file suit over forced abortions. 28 August.

Associated Press (2007) Portuguese abortion law approved CNN. www.aptn.80256FE9003E.F.444(httpstories) (accessed 14 July 2007).

Austveg B and Sundby J (2005) Norway at ICPD+10: International Assistance for reproductive health does not reflect domestic policies. *Reproductive Health Matters* 13(25): 233.

Babablu (2004) Cuba and Abortion Internet blog 11 Feb. www.babablu blog.com/archive/000458.html (accessed 17 July 2007).

Badgley RF, Caron M and Powell MG (1977) *Committee on the Operation of the Abortion Law.* Ministry of Supply and Services Canada: Ottawa.

Bailey PE, Bruno ZV, Bezerra MF, Queiroz I, Oliveira CM and Chen-Mok (2001) Adolescent pregnancy one year later: the effects of abortion vs. motherhood in Northeast Brazil. *Journal of Adolescent Health* 29: 223–32.

Bangladesh Bureau of Statistics (2000) *Abortion in Bangladesh.* Government of Bangladesh: Dhaka.

Berenstein N (2006a) *Abortion in Argentina.* Planned Parenthood: Washington DC.

Berenstein N (2006b) *Post-abortion Care in Argentina.* Planned Parenthood: Washington DC.

Berer M (2000) Making abortions safe: a matter of good public health policy and practice. *Bulletin of the World Health Organization* 78(5): 580–92. Available online at http://whqlibdoc.who.int/bulletin/2000/Number%205/78(5)5805–92.pdf (accessed 24 January 2007).

Berer M (2004) National laws and unsafe abortion; the parameters of change. *Reproductive Health Matters* 12(24): 1–9.

Berer M (2005) Why medical abortion is important to women. *Reproductive Health Matters* 13(26): 6–10.

Bhuiya A, Aziz A and Chowdhury M (2001) Ordeal for women of induced abortion in a rural area of Bangladesh. *Journal of Health Population and Nutrition* 19(4): 281–90.

Birkett WN (1939) *Report of the Inter-departmental Committee on Abortion*. HMSO: London.

Birth Rate Commission (1917) *The Declining Birth Rate*, 2nd edn. Chapman and Hall: London.

Bitler M and Zavodny M (2002) Did abortion legalization reduce the number of unwanted children? Evidence from adoptions. *Perspectives on Sexual and Reproductive Health* 34(1): 25–33.

Blanchard K, Winikoff B, Coyaji K et al. (2000) Misoprostol alone – a new method of medical abortion. *Journal of the American Medical Women's Association* 55: 189–90.

Blum W, Resnick MD and Stark TA (1987) The impact of a parental notification law on adolescent abortion decision making. *American Journal of Public Health* 77(5): 619–20.

BMA (2007) Ethics: *BMA Briefing Paper*. British Medical Association: London.

Bongaarts J (1997) Trends in unwanted childbearing in the developing world. *Studies in Family Planning* 28(4): 267–77.

Boonstra HD, Benson Gold R, Richards CL and Finer LB (2006) *Abortion in Women's Lives*. Guttmacher Institute: New York, p.4. Available online at http://www.guttmacher.org/pubs/2006/05/04/AiWL.pdf (accessed 10 May 2007).

Borgmann C and Weiss C (2003) Beyond apocalypse and apology: a moral defense of abortion. *Perspectives on Sexual and Reproductive Health* 35(1):40–3. Available online at http://www.guttmacher.org/pubs/journals/3504003.pdf (accessed 23 February 2007).

Bourque O (2006) Quebec told to reimburse women for abortions. *Globe and Mail*, 19 August.

Brodie JS, Gavigan AM and Jenson J (1992) *The Politics of Abortion*. Oxford University Press: Toronto.

Brookman Amissah E and Moyo JB (2004) Abortion Law Reform in Sub-Saharan Africa. *Reproductive Health Matters* 12(23): 2272–34.

Cabatu E and Bonk K (2005) Media Summary (Agency France Presse) 6 March. *Global population media analysis*. ncseonline.org/pop planet/ccmc/html/2000july15 (accessed 24 July 2007).

Calverton MD (2003) *Reproductive, Maternal and Child Health in Eastern Europe and Eurasia: a comparative report*. Macro International Inc.: Washington DC.

CAN/LW News (2007) Uruguay's new top judge backs abortion. *CAN/LW News.com*, 1 February.

Carbonell JLL, Varela L, Velazco A et al. (1997) The use of misoprostol for abortion at <9 weeks gestation. *European Journal of Contraceptive and Reproductive Health Care* 2: 181–5.

Cartoof VG and Klerman L V (1986) Parental consent for abortion: impact of the Massachusetts law. *American Journal of Public Health* 76(4): 397–400.

Catalinotti E (2007) Portugal. *Workers World*, 13 February.

Cates W Jr, Grimes DA and Shulz KF (2003) The public health impact of legal abortion: thirty years later. *Perspectives on Sexual and Reproductive Health* 35: 25–8.

*Catholic Encyclopaedia* (1913) Encyclopaedia Press: London, pp.44–50.

Catholic News Agency (2007) Pro-abortion senator plans new law. Montevideo, 9 January.

CBC (1998) Canadians firm on beliefs about abortion. CBC News, 13 November. www.cbc.ca (accessed 30 March 2007).

CBC (2004) Manitoba must pay for private abortions, judge rules. CBC News, 24 December. http://www.cbc.ca/canada/story/2004/12/24/abortion-041224.html (accessed 25 March 2007).

Center for Reproductive Rights (2005) *The World's Abortion Laws*. http://www.crlp.org/pub_fac_abortion_laws.html (accessed 15 Feb 2007).

Chakwe M (2007) Abortion in Zambia. *The Post* Newspaper, Zambia, 28 January.

Chavez S (2003) The gag rule from the perspective of the woman's movement in Peru: Briefing to US Congress 22 October. Published under the title *On the Hill*. US Congress: Washington DC.

Chelala C (1998) Algerian abortion controversy highlights rape of war victims. *Lancet* 351: 1413.

Chiarelli N (2004) More from southeast get abortions in the capital. *New Brunswick Telegraph Journal*, 12 January: (A3).

Childbirth by Choice Trust (1998) *No Choice: Canadian Women Tell their Stories of Illegal Abortion*. Childbirth by Choice Trust: Toronto.

Childbirth by Choice Trust (2007) *Abortion: Sweden*. Childbirth by Choice Trust: Toronto.

Chinoy M (2007) Vietnam's high abortion rate. *Medical News Today*, 18 February.

Choike (2002) *Women and Health in Uruguay*. Choike.org (accessed 10 Dec 2006).

Chrissman M, Moore R, Mondy L et al. (1980) Effects of restricting federal funds for abortion – Texas. *Morbidity and Mortality Weekly* 29(22): 253–4.

CIA (2007) *World Fact Book: Chile*. UN: New York.

Cliff E (2004) *March for Women's Lives*. Boloji.com (accessed 9 May 2007).

Conde CH (2005) Philippines Abortion Crisis. *International Herald Tribune*, 16 May.

Cook PJ, Parnell AM, Moore MJ and Pagnini D (1999) The effects of short-term variation in abortion funding on pregnancy outcomes *Journal of Health Economics* 18: 241–57.

Crane B and Hord C (2006) Access to safe abortion: an essential strategy for achieving the millennium development goals to improve maternal health, promote gender equality, and reduce poverty. Ipas: Chapel Hill. Available at http://www.unmillenniumproject.org/documents/Crane_and_Hord-Smith-final.pdf (accessed 9 May 2007).

CRR (2004) Safe and legal abortion is a woman's human right. CRR briefing paper: *What if Roe Fell? The State-by-state Consequences of Overturning Roe v Wade*. Center For Reproductive Rights: New York.

da Cunha e Tavora F (2007) Abortion. *The Economist*, 13 February.

Dagg PK (1991) The psychological sequelae of therapeutic abortion – denied and completed. *American Journal of Psychiatry* 148(5): 578–85.

da Silva WI (2003) *At Reproductive Health in Sri Lanka*. US AID.

de Bruijn J (1979) *Geschiedenis van Abortus in Nederland*. Van Gennep: Amsterdam.

de Bruijn B and Horstman R (2005) *Population and Abortion Activities*. http://www.resourceflows.org/index.php (accessed 13 June 2007).

DeJong J, Jawad J, Mortagy I and Shepard B (2005) The sexual and reproductive health of young people in the Arab countries and Iran. *Reproductive Health Matters* 13(25): 49–50.

de Jonge ETM, Pattison RC and Mantel GC (1999) Termination of pregnancy (TOP) in South Africa in its first year: is TOP getting on top of the problem of safe abortion? *Sexual and Reproductive Health Bulletin* 7: 14–15.

del Carmen Elu M (1993) Abortion yes, abortion no in Mexico. *Reproductive Health Matters* 1(1): 58–66.

de Sam Lazaro, F (2004) *Religion and Ethics* Newsletter.
www.pbs.org/newshour/bb/africa/janjune04Zambia.01-08html (accessed 9 January 2007).

Deschner A and Cohen SA (2003) Contraceptive use is key to reducing abortion. *Guttmacher Institute* 6(4): 7–10.

Dickens B (1991) Canada: abortion bill defeated. *Lancet* 337(8740): 543.

Dickson-Tetteh K and Rees H (1999) Efforts to reduce abortion related mortality in South Africa. In Beret M and Rawindran TK (eds.) *Safe Motherhood Initiatives: Critical Issues.* Blackwell Science: Oxford, pp.198–219.

Digest (1998) Yemen. *Family Planning Perspectives* 24(1).

Dunphy C (1996) *Morgentaler: A Difficult Hero*. Random House of Canada: Toronto.

Easton A (2007) Polish woman wins abortion case. BBC News Warsaw.
http://news.bbc.co.uk/1/hi/world/europe/6470403.stm (accessed 4 April 2007).

Egan JE, Benn PA, Zelop CM et al. (2004) Down syndrome births in the United States from 1989–2001. *American Journal of Obstetrics and Gynecology* 191(3): 1044–8.

Eggertson L (2001) Abortion services in Canada: a patchwork quilt with many holes. *Canadian Medical Association Journal* 164(6): 847.

Eisenberg D (2007) Abortion in Jewish law. *Society Today* Homepage: Aish.com.
www/societyworks/sciencenature/abin.j.law.asp (accessed 17 July 2007).

Elderton EM (1914) *Report on the English Birth Rate*. Eugenics Society: London.

Ellis HH (1933) *Psychology of Sex*. Heinemann: London.

Estrada D (2006) Chile: Therapeutic abortion a distant but not impossible prospect.
psnews.net/news.asp?idnews=34850 (accessed 17 July 2007).

Facer W (1978) Initial consequences of the 1977 New Zealand abortion law. *New Zealand Nursing Forum* 6(2): 91–2.

Fargues P (2005) Women in Arab countries: challenging the patriarchal system? *Reproductive Health Matters* 13(25): 43–8.

Faúndes A and Barzelatto JS (2006) *The Human Drama of Abortion. A Global Search for Consensus*. Vanderbilt University Press: Nashville.

Faúndes A, Duarte GA, Neto JA and de Sousa MH (2004) The closer you are, the better you understand: the reaction of Brazilian obstetrician-gynaecologists to unwanted pregnancy. *Reproductive Health Matters* 12(24): 47–56.

Fetter ST (2006) Abortion care needs in Darfur and Chad. *Forced Migration Review*, 3 May.

Finer LB, Frohwirth L, Dauphinee L, Singh S and Moore A (2005) Reasons US women have abortions: quantitative and qualitative perspectives. *Perspectives on Sexual and Reproductive Health* 37(3): 110–18.

Finer LB and Henshaw SK (2006) Disparities in the rate of unintended pregnancy in the United States 1994–2001. Perspectives on Sexual and Reproductive Health 38:2: 90–6.

Finney PA (1935) *Moral Problems in Hospital Practice*, 5th edn. B Herder: London.

Fisher W (2005) *Global Gag Rule* (24 Aug). http://www.commondreams.org/headlines05/0824-05.htm (accessed 17 July 2007).

Fonseca H and Pujol P (2004) A drama unfolds. *New Internationalist*, November.

FPASL (2000) Reduction of unplanned pregnancy and recourse to induced abortion, FPASL Seminar, 20–22 August.

Francome C (1976) How many illegal abortions? *British Journal of Criminology* 16(4): 389–92.

Francome C (1977) Estimating the number of illegal abortions. *Journal of Biosocial Science* 9: 467–9.

Francome C (1978) Abortion: why the issue has not disappeared. *Political Quarterly* 49(2): 217–22.

Francome C (1983) Unwanted pregnancies amongst teenagers. *Journal of Biosocial Science* 15(2).

Francome C (1984a) *Abortion Freedom*. Unwin Hyman: London.

Francome C (1984b) Historical view of the safe period. *Breaking Chains* n.d.

Francome C (1986) *Abortion Practice*. Unwin Hyman: London.

Francome C (2004) *Abortion in the USA and the UK*. Ashgate Publishing: Aldershot.

Fuchs D (2005) Spanish abortion rate soars. *Guardian*, 28 December.

Gallo MF, Gebreselassie H, Victorino MTA et al. (2004) Assessment of abortion services in public health facilities in Mozambique: women's and provider's perspectives. *Reproductive Health Matters* 12(24): 218–26.

Ganatra B, Bygdeman M, Thuy PB et al. (2004) From research to reality: the challenges of introducing medical abortion into service delivery in Vietnam. *Reproductive Health Matters* 12(24): 105–13.

Garcia SG, Tatum C, Becker D et al. (2004) Policy implication of a national public opinion survey on abortion in Mexico. *Reproductive Health Matters* 12(24): 65–74.

Genethique (2005) www.genethique.org (accessed 14 July 2007).

Global Health Council (2002) *Promises to Keep: The Toll of Unintended Pregnancies on Women's Lives in the Developing World*. Global Health Council: Washington DC.

Global News (2005) UNICEF report: Children and Women's Rights in Zimbabwe, 30 March 2005.

Goldman LA, Garcia SG, Diaz J and Yan EA (2005) Brazil, obstetricians and gynecologists and abortion. *Reproductive Health Matters* 15 Nov(2):10.

Gordon L (1977) *Women's Body, Women's Right*. Penguin: Harmondsworth.

Grimes DA (1999) Estimation of pregnancy-related mortality risk by pregnancy outcome. United States 1991–99. *American Journal of Obstetrics and Gynecology* 194:92–4.

Grimes DA, Benson J, Singh S et al. (2006) *Unsafe Abortion the Preventable Pandemic*. www.medicalnewstoday.com/articles/55593php (accessed 17 July 2007).

Grossman M and Jacobowitz S (1981) Variation in infant mortality rates among counties of the United States: the roles of public policies and programs. *Demography* 18(4): 695–713.

*Guardian* (2007) US doubles help for aids programmes. 31 May.

Gumbel A (2006) Colombia ruling breaks seal on abortion. *Independent*, 13 May.

Guttmacher Institute (1999) *Sharing Responsibilities: Women, Society and Abortion Worldwide*. Guttmacher Institute: New York.

Guttmacher Institute (2006) *State Policies in Brief: State Funding of Abortion Under Medicaid*. Org/statecenter/spibs/spib_SFAM.pdf (accessed 16 May 2006).

Guttmacher S, Kapadia F, te Water Naude J and de Pinho H (1998) Abortion law reform in South Africa: a case study of the 1996 Choice on Termination of Pregnancy Act. *International Family Planning Perspectives* 24(4).

Hajnal J (1965) A comparison of family patterns in Eastern and Western Europe. In Glass DV and Eversley DEC (eds.) *Population in History*. Metheun: London.

Hale EM (1860) On the homeopathic treatment of abortion. In Francome C *Abortion Practice*. Unwin Hyman: London.

Hall KG (2003) Abortion in Brazil: a debate divided along moral and class lines. *Knight Ridden Newspapers*, 28 July.

Halperin M (2007) *Termination of Pregnancy: Legal, Moral and Jewish Aspects*. Shaare Zedek: Jerusalem.

Health Canada (2002) *Canadian Health Act Overview*. http://www.hc-sc.gc.ca/ahc-asc/media/nr-cp/2002/2002_care-soinsbk4_e.html (accessed 30 March 2007).

Hennesy M and Smyth J (2007) European court ruling in Polish abortion case can affect the law here. *Irish Times*, 21 March.

Henriques A, Lourenço A, Ribeirinho A, Ferreira H and Graça L (2007) Maternal death related to misoprostol overdose. *Obstetrics and Gynecology* 109(2, part 2): 489–90.

Henshaw SK (1995) The impact of requirement for parental consent on minors' abortions in Mississippi. *Family Planning Perspectives* 27(3): 120–2.

Henshaw SK and Kost K (1992) Parental involvement in minors' abortion decisions. *Family Planning Perspectives* 24(5): 196–207, 213.

Henshaw SK, Singh S, Oye-Adeniran BO et al. (1998) The incidence of abortion in Nigeria. *Journal of International Family Planning Perspectives* 24(3): December.

Henshaw SK, Singh S and Hass T (1999) The incidence of abortion worldwide. *Family Planning Perspectives* 25(Suppl.): January.

Henshaw SK, Haas T, Berentsen K and Carbonne E (2001) *Readings on Induced Abortion, Vol. 2. A world review 2000*. Guttmacher Institute: New York.

Hessini L (2005) Global Progress in abortion advocacy and policy: an assessment of the decade since ICPD. *Reproductive Health Matters* 13(25): 88–100.

Hilgers TW and O'Hare D (1981) Abortion related maternal mortality: an in depth analysis. In Hilgers et al. (eds.) *New Perspecitves on Human Abortion*. University Publications of America Inc.: Frederick, Maryland, pp.69–91.

Hirve SS (2004) Abortion law, policy and services in India: a critical review. *Reproductive Health Matters* 12(24): 114–21.

Hodge HL (1854) *Criminal Abortion*. TK and PG Collins: New York.

Hollick F (1849) *Diseases of Women, their Causes and Cures Familiarly Explained*. TW Strong: New York.

Hovorun TV and Vornyk BM (2003) Ukraine, in *The International Encyclopedia of Sexuality*, Vol 6. Continuum: New York.

Human Rights Watch (2005) *Help for the Victims* hrw.org/reports/2005/drc0305/8 (accessed 17 July 2007).

Human Rights Watch (2007a) Obstacles to the right to decide in matters relating to abortion in Argentina. hrw.org/women/argentina (accessed 17 July 2007).

Human Rights Watch (2007b) Women's rights: Chile.hrw.org. (accessed 17 July 2007).

Human Rights Watch (2007c) Women's rights: Colombia.hrw.org/English/docs/2005/6/22/colomb (accessed 17 July 2007).

Human Rights Watch (2007d) Mexico: Rape victims denied legal abortion rights. hrw.org/English/docs/2006/2/23/mexico (accessed 17 July 2007).

Illingworth B (2006) Mexico's abortion law. Planned Parenthood of USA. www.pp.org//politics-policy-issues/internatonal-issues/mexico-abortion-13045.ntm (accessed 24 July 2007).

International Planned Parenthood Federation (IPPF) (2006) *Understanding Religious and Political Opposition to Sexual and Reproductive Health and Rights in Europe*. IPPF, European Network: Brussels.

International Women's Health Coalition (2007) Abortion in Peru. nytimes/gst/fullpage.html?res9D00E1DF (accessed 17 July 2007).

Ioannidi-Kapolou E (2004) Use of contraception and abortion in Greece: a review. *Reproductive Health Matters* 12(24): 174–83.

Jagwe-Wadda G, Moore AM and Wong V (2006) *Abortion Morbidity in Uganda*. Guttmacher Institute: New York.

Jahani F (2004) Abortion in Iranian law. Iran Daily Newspaper, 15 January.

Jewkes R, Rees H, Dickson K, Brown H and Levin J (2005) The impact of age on the epidemiology of incomplete abortions in South Africa after legislative change. *British Journal of Obstetrics and Gynaecology* 112(3): 355–9.

Johansen S (2004) *Who are the crisis pregnancy centres?* http://www.prochoiceactionnetwork-canada.org/articles/who-are-cpcs.shtml (accessed 10 July 2007).

Johnson BR, Horga M and Fajans P (2004) A strategic assessment of abortion and contraception in Romania. *Reproductive Health Matters* 12(24): 184–94.

Johnston WR (2005) *Swedish abortion rates by county 1998–2004.* www.johnstonsarchive.net/policy/abortion/sweden/ab-5wac2.html (accessed 17 July 2007).

Johnston WR (2007a) *Historical Abortion Statistics of Russia* (updated 20 Jan). www.johnstonsarchive.net/policy/abortion/-ab-russia.html (accessed 17 July 2007).

Johnston WR (2007b) *Historical Abortion Statistics of Israel.* www.johnstonsarchive,net/policy/abortion/-ab-israel.html (accessed 17 July 2007).

Johnston WR (2007c) *Historical Abortion Statistics of Saudi Arabia.* www.johnstonsarchive,net/policy/abortion/-ab-saudiarabia.html (accessed 17 July 2007).

Johnston WR (2007d) *Historical Abortion Statistics of Uzbekistan.* www.johnstonsarchive,net/policy/abortion/-ab-uzbekistan.html (accessed 17 July 2007).

Johnston WR (2007e) *Historical Abortion Statistics of Vietnam.* www.johnstonsarchive,net/policy/abortion/-ab-vietnam.html (accessed 17 July 2007).

Jones RK, Darroch JE and Henshaw SK (2002) Patterns in the socioeconomic characteristics of women obtaining abortions in 2000–2001. *Perspectives on Sexual and Reproductive Health* 34(5): 226–35.

Joyce T (1987) The impact of induced abortion on black and white birth outcomes in the United States. *Demography* 24(2): 229–44.

Joyce T, Kaestner R and Coleman S (2006) Change in abortion and births and the Texas parental notification law. *New England Journal of Medicine* 354(10): 1031–8.

Juaraz F, Cabigon J, Singh S and Hussain R (2005) The incidence of induced abortion in the Philippines. *International Family Planning Perspectives* 31(3): September.

Katzive L (2007) *Law Changes 1996–2007.* Center for Reproductive Rights: New York.

Ketting E and Schnabel P (1980) Induced abortion in the Netherlands: a decade of experience 1970–80. *Studies in Family Planning* 11(12): 385–94.

Kissling F (2006) *A Roman Catholic Defense for Decriminalizing Abortion*. Catholics for a Free Choice: Washington DC.

Kitamura K (2005) Abortion. *Japan's Mental Health*, 6 November.

Kommers DP (1977) Abortion and the Constitution: United States and West Germany. *American Journal of Comparative Law* 25(2): 225–85.

Konje JC, Obisesan KA and Ladipo AO (1992) Health and economic consequences of septic induced abortion. *International Journal of Gynecology and Obstetrics* 37(3): 193–7.

Koopersmith TB and Mishell DR (1996) The use of misoprostol for termination of early pregnancy. *Contraception* 53: 237.

Ladipo OA (1989) Preventing and managing complications of induced abortion in third world countries. *International Journal of Gynecology and Obstetrics* 3(Suppl.): 21–8.

Lafaurie MM , Grossman D, Troncoso E, Billings DL and Chavez S (2005) Women's perspectives on medical abortion in Mexico, Columbia, Ecuador and Peru: a qualitative study. *Reproductive Health Matters* 13(26): 75–83.

Lak D (2002) Nepalese women win abortion rights. BBC News, 27 September.

Lane SD, Jok JM and El-Mouelhy MT (1998) Buying safety: the economics of reproductive risk and abortion in Egypt. *Social Science and Medicine* 47(8): 1089–99.

Langer A, Garcia-Barrios C, Heimburger A, Campero L, Stein K, Winikoff B and Barahona V (1999) Improving post-abortion care with limited resources in a public hospital in Oaxaca, Mexico. In Huntington D and Piet-Pelon NJ (eds.) *Post-abortion Care: Lessons from Operations Research*. Population Council New York: New York, pp.80–1.

Larijani B and Zahedi F (2006) Changing parameters for abortion in Iran. *Journal of Medical Ethics*. globalbioethics.blogspot.com/2007_03_01archive.html (accessed 17 July 2007).

Lerdmaleewong M and Francis C (1998) Abortion in Thailand: a feminist perspective. *Journal of Buddhist Ethics* 5: 22–48.

Levine PB, Staiger D, Kane TJ and Zimmerman DJ (1999) Roe v Wade and American Fertility. *American Journal of Public Health* 89(2): 199–203.

Life Site News (2003) Muslims approve cloning in Malaysia. www.lifesite.net/idn/2003/jan (accessed 4 April 2007).

Life Site News (2005) Spanish abortion rate doubles over 10 years. www.lifesite.net/idn/2005/feb/05021110.html (accessed 4 April 2007).

Linner B (1968) *Sex and Society in Sweden*. Cape: London.

Liskin LS (1992) Maternal morbidity in developing countries: a review and comments. *International Journal of Gynecology and Obstetrics* 37(2): 77–87.

Lusiola G (2005) *Hearing Women's Cries*. www.engender health.org/new-tanzania/whats new/iwdo5.html (accessed 17 July 2007).

McCracken M (2002) Manitoba women have access to abortions as long as they have time or money. *Canadian Centre for Policy Alternatives*: Fast Facts, September 23.

McLaren A and McLaren MT (1997) The Bedroom and the State: *The Changing Practices and Politics of Contraception and Abortion in Canada*, 1880–1997, 2nd edn. Oxford University Press: Toronto.

Majaj Y (ed.) (2005) *Ten Years after Beijing*. Arab NGOs UN Development Fund.

Matejcek Z, Dytrych Z and Schüller V (1985) Follow-up study of children born to women denied abortion. In *Ciba Foundation Symposium 115. Abortion: medical progress and social implications*. Pitman: London, pp.136–49.

Meaney J (2003) A Pro life Missionary trip. *Human Life International* November: 101–3.

Methodist Church (2003) Untitled statement on the position of the Church in Uruguay, released 3 February.

Micklewright J and Stewart K (1999) Austria UNICEF. Expert group meeting on policy responses to population. Population Division Department Economic and Social Affairs UN: New York.

Ministére de la Sante (2003) *Division de la Sante Familiale*. University of Lome.

Ministry of Health (2002) *Ethiopian Health and Health Related Indicators*. Ministry of Health: Addis Ababa.

Mohagheghpour S (1997) The Gag rule and Tanzania. www.plannedparenthood.org/.../politics-issues/international-issue/Tanzania-gag6461.htm (accessed 17 July 2007).

Mohr JC (1978) *Abortion in America*. Oxford University Press: Oxford.

Montesinos L and Preciado J (1997) Abortion: Puerto Rico *International Journal of Sexuality.* Available at www.sex quest.com//esa/iesi-3contents.html (accessed 17 July 2007).

Moore T (2003) *On Board Poland's Abortion Ship.* BBC Wladyslawowo.

Mpangile GS, Leshabari MT and Kihwele DJ (1993) Factors associated with induced abortion in public hospitals in Dar es Salaam, Tanzania. *Reproductive Health Matters* 1(2): 21–31.

MSI (2007a) *Sri Lanka.* Marie Stopes International: London.

MSI (2007b) *Tanzania.* Marie Stopes International: London.

MSI (2007c) *Uganda: Providing a Life Guard against HIV.* Marie Stopes International: London.

Mturi AJ and Hinde A (2001) *Fertility Levels and Differentials in Tanzania.* www.un.org/esa/populationpublications/prospects decline info3.pdf (accessed 17 July 2007).

Muldoon M (1991) *The Abortion Debate in the United States and Canada: A Source Book.* Garland: New York.

Mundigo A and Indriso C (1999) *Abortion in the Developed World.* Zed Books: London.

Myers SL (2003) After decades: Russia narrows grounds for abortion. *New York Times,* 24 August.

Nowicka W (2005) Contemporary women's hell: Polish women's stories. *Reproductive Health Matters* 13(26): 160–4.

Nunes FE and Delph YM (1997) Making abortion reform work: steps and slips in Guyana. *Reproductive Health Matters* 9: 66–76.

Olori T (2007) Abortion Law takes a toll. *International Press News Agency,* 15 February.

Osofsky HJ and Osofsky JD (1973) *The Abortion Experience.* Harper and Row: London.

Ottoway M (2004) *Women's Rights and Democracy in the Arab World.* Carnegie Papers: Washington DC.

Page J (2007a) Vibrating condoms attacked by Hindus as illicit 'sex toys'. *The Times,* 20 June: 34 col 2.

Page J (2007b) Hospital mass grave found as India cracks down on female infanticide. *The Times,* 19 February(Section 1): 27 col 1.

Palley HA (2006) Canadian abortion policy: national policy and the impact of federalism and political implementation on access to services. *Publius: The Journal of Federalism* 36(4): 565–86.

Palmdoc (2006) Should abortion be legalized in Malaysia? *Malayan Medical Resources.* http/www.medicine.com.my/wp/wp-mobile.php?p=13288more=1 (accessed 17 July 2007).

Pangkahila W and Pangkahila JA (2006) *Indonesia.* www2.hu-berlin.de.sexology/IES/Indonesia-part1.html (accessed 17 July 2007).

Parish TN (1935) A thousand cases of abortion. *Journal of Obstetrics and Gynaecology of the British Empire* 1107.

Parry LA (1932) *Criminal Abortion.* Bale Press: London.

Paulson KD (2007) *Seventh Day Adventists: Abortion* (accessed 17 April 2007).

Paxman JM (1980) *Law and Planned Parenthood.* IPPF: London.

Pelrine VW (1972) *Abortion in Canada.* New Press: Toronto.

Perlez J (2007) Warsaw bans a clinic's in vitro fertilization treatments. *New York Times,* 3 April.

Perner RA (2007) *Austria.* Reputik Osterreich International Encyclopedia of Sexuality. www2.hu-berlin.de/sexology/IES/Austria.html (accessed 17 July 2007).

Pheterson G and Azize Y (2005) Abortion practice in the northeast Caribbean: Just write down stomach pain. *Reproductive Health Matters* 13(26): 44–53.

Phillips B (1999) Maternal deaths take a heavy toll in Nigeria. BBC News, 26 June.

Population Division (2007a) *Abortion Policy: Thailand*. Department of Economic and Social Affairs UN: New York.

Population Division (2007b) *Abortion Policy: Turkey*. Department of Economic and Social Affairs UN: New York.

Population Division (2007c) *Abortion Policy: Uzbekistan*. Department of Economic and Social Affairs UN: New York.

Population Division (2007d) *Abortion Policy: Yemen*. Department of Economic and Social Affairs UN: New York.

Population Division (2007e) *Abortion Policy: Nigeria*. Department of Economic and Social Affairs UN: New York.

Population Division (2007f) *Abortion Policy: Tanzania*. Department of Economic and Social Affairs UN: New York.

Population Division (2007g) *Abortion Policy: Zambia*. Department of Economic and Social Affairs UN: New York.

Population Division (2007h) *Abortion Policy: Venezuela*. Department of Economic and Social Affairs UN: New York.

Population Information Program (2007) Center for Communication Programs, Vol. 25 No. 1. The Johns Hopkins School of Public Health: Baltimore.

Population Reference Bureau (2007) *Turkey: Abortion*. International Woman's Health Coalition: Washington DC.

Potts M, Diggory P and Peel J (1977) *Abortion*. Cambridge University Press: Cambridge.

Pratt M and Werchick L (2004) *Sexual Terrorism: Rape as a Weapon*. US/AID/DCHA: Washington DC.

Rahman A, Katzive L and Henshaw SK (1998) A global review of laws on induced abortion, 1985–1987. *International Family Planning Perspectives* 24(2): 56–64.

Rasch V and Lyaruu MA (2005) Unsafe abortion in Tanzania: the need for involving men in post-abortion counselling. *Family Planning Perspectives* 36(4): 201–10.

Rees H, Katzenellenbogen J, Shabodien R, Jewkes R, Fawcus S, McIntyre J, Lombard C and Truter H (1997) The epidemiology of incomplete abortion in South Africa. *South African Medical Journal* 87(4): 432–7.

Religion and Ethics (2004) Newsletter: Zambia, 9 January.

Religious Tolerance (2005) *Abortion News* (accessed 17 July 2007).

Reynolds M (2005) Abortion rate drops to lowest ever. *The Oregue Post*, 27 July.

RF (Resources Flow) News (2004) *Briefing September*, from UNFPA/UNAIDS and NIDO (Netherlands Interdisciplinary Demographic Institute).

RF (Resources Flow) News (2007) *Briefing March,* from UNFPA/UNAIDS and NIDO (Netherlands Interdisciplinary Demographic Institute).

Rodgers S (2006) Abortion denied: bearing the limits of the law, in C Flood (ed.) *Just Medicare: What's in, What's out, How we Decide*. University of Toronto Press: Toronto, pp.107–36.

Rogers JL, Boruch RF, Stoms GB et al. (1991) Impact of the Minnesota parental notification law on abortion and birth. *American Journal of Public Health* 81(3): 294–8.

Rongy AJ (1933) *Abortion Legal or Illegal*. Vanguard: New York.

Ross J (2005) *Illegal abortion rampant in Latin America*. Women's News. www.womensenews.org.article.cfm/dyn/aid2086/context/archive (accessed 17 July 2007).

Ross J (2006) *Chile's teens sex health.* Women's News. www.womensenews.org/article.cfm/dyn/aid/2895/context/archive (accessed 17 July 2007).

Rossier C, Guielle G, Ouédraogo A and Thiéba B (2004) Estimating clandestine abortion with the confidants method. Results from Ouagadougou, Burkina Faso. Paper presented at the Population Association of America, April. http://paa2004.princeton.edu/download.asp?submissionId=41577 (accessed 31 January 2006).

Round Up (2005a) Health and health services suffering in Iraq. *Reproductive Health Matters* 13: 190.

Round Up (2005b) Improving reproductive health services in Pakistan. *Reproductive Health Matters* 13: 191.

Royal Commission (1977) *Contraception, sterilization and abortion in New Zealand.* NZ Government Publication: Auckland.

St John Stevas N (1963) *The Right to Life.* Hodder and Stoughton: London.

Sanger M (1938) *My Fight for Birth Control.* WW Norton: New York.

Schuster S (2005) Abortion in the moral world of the grassfields of Cameroon. *Reproductive Health Matters* 13(26): 130–8.

Secretary General (2005) *Financial Research Flow for Population Advice in 2004.* UN: New York.

Senlet P, Cagatay L and Matthis J (2001) Bridging the gap: integrating family planning with abortion services in Turkey. *International Journal of Family Planning* 27(2): June.

Shakya G, Kishore S, Bird C and Barak J (2004) Abortion law reform in Nepal: women's right to life and health. *Reproductive Health Matters* 12(24): 75–84.

Shaw J (2007) *Reality Check: A close look at accessing abortion services in Canadian hospitals.* Canadians for Choice. Available at: www.canadiansforchoice.ca (accessed 5 April 2007).

Singh S (2006) Hospital admissions resulting from unsafe abortion: estimates from 13 developing countries. Lancet 368: 1887–92.

Singh S, Darroch J, Vlassof M and Nadeau J (2003) *Adding it up: the Benefits of Investing in Sexual and Reproductive Health Care.* Guttmacher Institute: New York.

Singh Y (2004) Abortion nightmare in Nepal. BBC News. News.bbc.co.uk/2/hi/south_asia/397/127.stm (accessed 16 Feb 2007).

Smith D (2003) *The Atlas of War and Peace.* Earthscan and CIA: Washington DC.

Statistics Canada (2003) 2001 Census: *Analysis Series, Religions in Canada.* Minister of Industry. Catalogue no. 96F0030XIE2001015. Available at: www.statcan.ca (accessed 31 July 2007).

Statistics Canada (2006) Induced abortions, 2003. *The Daily,* 15 March. Available at: www.statcan.ca (accessed 31 July 2007).

Statistics Canada (2007a) Portrait of the Canadian population in 2006, *2006 Census.* Minister of Industry. Statistics Canada Catalogue no.975–50-XIE. Available at: www.statcan.ca (accessed 31 July 2007).

Statistics Canada (2007b) Induced abortions by area of residence of patients. CANSIM Table 106–9013, Catalogue no. 822–23-XIE. Available at: www.statcan.ca (accessed 31 July 2007).

Steel C and Chiarotti S (2004) With everything exposed: cruelty in post-abortion care in Rosario, Argentina. *Reproductive Health Matters* 12(24): 39–46.

Stephenson P, Wagner M, Badea M and Serbanescu F (1992) Commentary: the public health consequences of restricted induced abortion. Lessons from Romania. *American Journal of Public Health* 82(10): 1328–31.

Stone L (1977) *The family, sex and marriage in England 1500–1800.* Weidenfeld and Nicholson: London.

Storer HR (1866) *Why Not? A Book for Every Woman.* Lee and Shepard: New York.

Strauss LT, Herndon J, Chang J, Parker W, Bowens S, Zane S and Berg C. (2004) Abortion surveillance – United States Centers for Disease Control and Prevention. *Surveillance Summaries,* 26 Nov: 53 (no SS-9).

Susser M (1992) Induced abortion and health as a value. *American Journal of Public Health* 82(10): 1323–4.

Szczech K (2007) Polish women to Sweden for abortion. www.polish.youth.org (accessed 17 May 2007).

Takeshita YJ, Tan Boon A and Arshat H (1986) Attitudes towards induced abortion. *Malay Journal of Reproductive Health* December (2): 73–90.

Taussig FJ (1910) *Prevention and Treatment of Abortion.* CV Mosby: St Louis.

Taussig FJ (1936) *Abortion – Spontaneous and Induced.* CV Mosby: St Louis.

Thapa S (2004) Abortion law in Nepal: the road to reform. *Reproductive Health Matters* 12(24): 85–94.

Tietze C (1984) The public health effects of legal abortion in the United States. *Family Planning Perspectives* 16(1): 26–8.

Tietze C, Pakter J and Berger TS (1972) Mortality with legal abortion in New York City, 1970– 1972. *Journal of the American Medical Association* 225(5): 507–9.

Toussa-Ahossu A (1991) *Contribution a l'ètude de la mortalité maternalle dans deux materternités urbaines du Toga.* University of Benin: Lome.

Treffers PE (1965) Abortus en Anticonceptie. Bohn: Haarlem.

Trussell J, Menken J, Lindheim B and Vaughan B (1980) The impact of restricting Medicaid financing for abortion. *Family Planning Perspectives* 12(3): 120–30.

UN (1995) Report of the International Conference On Population And Development. Cairo, September 5–13, 1994. UN: New York.

UN (1998) Summary Record of Meeting 1683, 28 July. UN: New York.

UN (2002) *Ukraine.* UN: New York.

UN (2003) *Yemen.* UN: New York.

UN (2004) *World Population Monitoring.* UN: New York.

UN (2006) *Korea South.* UN: New York.

UN (2007) Decisions denied: women's access to contraception and abortion in Argentina. hrw.org/women/argentina (accessed 17 July 2007).

United Press International (2007) www.upi.com (accessed 17 July 2007).

Uprety A (1998) Abortion Laws in Nepal. *Body Politic* 8(3).

USA Bureau of Democracy (2001) *Saudi Arabia.* USA Bureau of Democracy: Washington.

Vekemans M and de Silva U (2005) HIV positive women and their right to choose. *Entre Nous* 59: 17–19.

Ventura SJ (2004) Estimating pregnancy rates for the United States 1990–2000. *National Vital Statistics. Reports.* 15 June 52(23).

Vieira C (2005) Columbia: Magistrates for partially lifting the abortion ban. International Press Service News Agency. /ipsnews.net/news.asp?idnews=33214 (accessed 11 May 2007).

Wainer B (1972) *Isn't it nice?* Aplan Books: Sydney.

Ward L (2007a) Abortions increase by 4% in one year. *Guardian*, 20 June.

Ward L (2007b) MPs to consider cut in abortion time limit. *Guardian*, 21 June.

Webb S (2000) *Addressing the Consequences of Unsafe Abortion*. Pathfinder International: Watertown, MA.

Wente M (2004) Abortion: the Tories other flashpoint. *Globe and Mail,* 3 June: A21.

Westen JH (2006a) Pope: abortion never. Life Site News.com, 21 September. www.lifesite.net/idn/2006/may/06050311.html (accessed 3 May 2007).

Westen JH (2006b) Sri Lankan pro life group stirs emotions with prayers outside abortion centre. www.lifesite.net/idn/2006/may/06050311.html (accessed 3 May 2007).

White H (2006) *Chile's Legislature soundly rejects abortion.* www.lifesite.net/idn/2006/nov/06112209.html (accessed 3 May 2007).

Whittaker A (2002) Abortion policy and practice. *Women and Health* 35: 4.

Whittaker A (2003) *Abortion Law Reform Advocacy in Thailand*. Palgrave Macmillan: London.

Whittaker A (2004) *Abortion, Sin and the State in Thailand*. Routledge, Chapman and Hall: London.

WHO (1999) *Abortion in Vietnam*. WHO: Geneva.

WHO (2002) *Estimates of DALYs by Sex, Cause and WHO Mortality Sub-region, Estimates for 2001*. WHO: Geneva.

WHO (2004) *Unsafe Abortion. Global and Regional Estimates of the Incidence of Unsafe Abortion and Associated Mortality in 2000*, 4th edn. WHO: Geneva.

WHO (2006) South East Asia Region Office: *Country Fact File on Maternal, Newborn and Child Health Situation in Indonesia* http://w3.whosea.org/en/section260/section1808/section1935/section1939_9149.htm (accessed January 2006).

WHO (2007) *European Health for All Database* http://www.euro.who.int/hfadb (accessed 10 May 2007).

WHO Forum (2006) Global Abortion News Update, 7 December (accessed 4 March 2007).

Woodside M (1963) Attitudes of women abortionists. *Howard Journal* 11: 93.

Wright JW (2006) 2007: *The New York Times Almanac*. Penguin: New York.

Xinhua (2004) China bans selective abortion to fix imbalance. www.chinadaily.com.cn/china/2006/8/8 content_660041.htm (accessed 16 July 2007).

# Index

# Other Titles in the **Middlesex University Press Health Series**

### Birth and Power
A Savage Enquiry Revisited
**Wendy Savage**
ISBN 978 1 904750 58 1/1 904750 58 3
Price £25

*Birth and Power – A Savage Enquiry Revisited* examines the issue of academic freedom, with particular reference to the medical profession and addresses the question of who controls childbirth. Contributions include a woman surgeon's personal account of suspension from practice; an account of the threats to academic freedom from an academic who blew the whistle and suffered the consequences and a discussion on accountability by the esteemed professor, James Drife. *Birth and Power* will be of interest to academics, health workers, social researchers, teachers, students and mothers. *Birth and Power* contains the complete text of *A Savage Enquiry*.

### Caesarean Birth in Britain:
### Revised and Updated
A book for health professionals and parents
**Wendy Savage, Helen Churchill,**
**Colin Francome**
ISBN 978 1 904750 17 8 / 1 904750 17 6
Price £18

*Caesarean Birth in Britain* presents expectant parents, educators and health professionals with the facts and figures, and documents a number of important changes which have occurred in obstetrics since the original book was published in 1993. Using data from a nationwide survey of obstetricians, the authors offer a comprehensive analysis of what has changed and ask at what cost.

### Vaginal Birth After Caesarean
The VBAC handbook
**Helen Churchill and Wendy Savage**
ISBN 978 1 904750 21 5
Price £6.99

*Vaginal Birth After Caesarean* presents pregnant women and health professionals with all the necessary information regarding options for birth following caesarean delivery. The handbook provides suggestions for constructive ways to achieve vaginal birth after caesarean (VBAC) when this is the right option. The book includes several successful VBAC stories.

### How to Avoid an Unnecessary Caesarean
A handbook for women who want a natural birth
**Helen Churchill and Wendy Savage**
ISBN 978 1 904750 16 1
Price £6.99

*How to Avoid an Unnecessary Caesarean* is aimed mainly at pregnant women and health professionals. The book provides case studies and suggestions for constructive ways to avoid unnecessary caesareans.

## Health Policy Reform: Driving the Wrong Way?

A Critical Guide to the Global 'Health Reform' Industry

**John Lister**

ISBN 978 1 904750 45 1 / 1 904750 45 1

Price £25

*Health Policy Reform: Driving the Wrong Way?* focuses on the main structural, managerial and policy changes that have been taking place within the world's health care systems since the early 1990s. It questions whether these 'reforms' are driven primarily by the health needs of the wider population or, in fact, by non-health considerations – the financial, ideological and political concerns of governments and global institutions. This text contains up-to-date facts and case studies making this a valuable reference work on health care reform and health policy.

## Female Genital Mutilation

Treating the Tears

**Haseena Lockhat**

ISBN 978 1 898253 90 7 / 1 898253 90 0

Price £15.99

*Female Genital Mutilation: Treating the Tears* deals with the topical and controversial issue of female circumcision. A thoroughly researched and academic work, it aims to raise awareness not only of the physical but also the psychological effects of this procedure. Female Genital Mutilation (FGM) has re-surfaced in the UK since the 1980s following the migration of people from FGM-practising countries. Various professionals nationwide are likely to encounter girls and women who have been either circumcised or are 'at risk' of being circumcised, as such this is a useful reference for those working in the health and social care industry.

**Ordering Information**

To order any of the above titles, please visit **www.mupress.co.uk**